PRAISE FOR *ALCHEMICAL HEALING*

"Nicky Scully presents a detaile⋯⋯⋯⋯⋯rans-
formational practices from the e⋯⋯⋯⋯. wise
and wonderful book to be savo⋯⋯⋯ great benefits to
those who practice and apply these methods."

RALPH METZNER, PH.D., PSYCHOLOGIST,
AUTHOR OF *THE UNFOLDING SELF*

"Artist, philosopher, traveler, alchemist, and healer, Nicki Scully has
healed herself and brought the light of healing to everyone around
her. *Alchemical Healing* is rich and whole-hearted, practical and
inspiring. I could not put it down."

ALBERTO VILLOLDO, PH.D.,
AUTHOR OF *SHAMAN, HEALER, SAGE*

"A lifetime of wisdom breathes inside these pages. If you could read
a book that would change and charge and heal your life, wouldn't
you? Nicki Scully has the Rx. She's got the mojo. This is the book."

NORMANDI ELLIS,
AUTHOR OF *AWAKENING OSIRIS:*
THE EGYPTIAN BOOK OF THE DEAD

"Here is a masterful work that provides clear instructions as to once
and future ways of healing self, other, and planet. Here is alchemy
at its best and most comprehensive. The reader is charged with
delight in new possibilities growing out of ancient knowings. Scully
gives us a book that is to be savored as well as used."

JEAN HOUSTON, PH.D.,
AUTHOR OF *JUMP TIME* AND *A MYTHIC LIFE*

"Nicki Scully is one of most innovative healers on the planet. In
Alchemical Healing, she shares what she has learned about physical
and spiritual transformation and includes excercises, meditations, and
visualizations that serve to put the information to immediate use.

STANLEY KRIPPNER, PH.D., CO-AUTHOR OF
EXTRAORDINARY DREAMS AND HOW TO USE THEM

"*Alchemical Healing* is a living bridge to ancient wisdom, a golden gift to all who would begin the Great Work of personal and global transformation. Using the terminology and operations of alchemy, Nicki Scully presents a bona fide and universal system of initiation and healing."

DENNIS WILLIAM HAUCK, ALCHEMIST AND AUTHOR OF
THE EMERALD TABLET:
ALCHEMY FOR PERSONAL TRANSFORMATION

"Nicki Sully's *Alchemical Healing* is a welcome addition to Chopra's *Quantum Healing* and deals specifically and forcibly with new insights based on ancient wisdom on just what you need to do to let the healing process occur."

FRED ALAN WOLF, PH.D.,
AUTHOR OF *MATTER INTO FEELING:*
A NEW ALCHEMY OF SCIENCE AND SPIRIT

"High praise for Nicki and this excellent book! Nicki, herself a healed-healer, brings to this offering her experience, wisdom, and personal passion for creatively addressing all forms of dis-ease, along with a fierce dedication to supporting others in the process of awakening and developing their healing hearts and hands. This is a powerful and timely book that supports resolution of the challenging issues of our time through our own offering of healing to All Our Relations."

BROOKE MEDICINE EAGLE,
AUTHOR OF *BUFFALO WOMAN COMES SINGING* AND
THE LAST GHOST DANCE

"Nicki Scully may well be one of the great alchemical practitioners of our time. A medical intuitive, teacher, and healer, in *Alchemical Healing* she shares her own fascinating healing journey, then in step-by-step journeys, initiations, and exercises, provides readers with the tools necessary for using this ancient system of healing. A truly remarkable book that enables the reader to not only understand but to practice alchemical healing."

ROSEMARY GLADSTAR, HERBALIST,
AUTHOR OF *HERBAL HEALING FOR WOMAN* AND
FOUNDER OF UNITED PLANT SAVERS

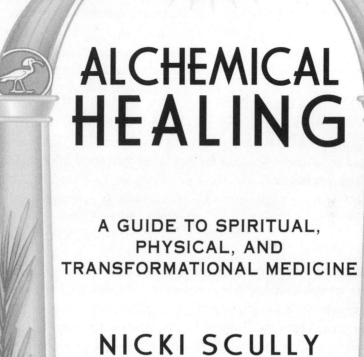

ALCHEMICAL
HEALING

A GUIDE TO SPIRITUAL, PHYSICAL, AND TRANSFORMATIONAL MEDICINE

NICKI SCULLY

Illustrated by
Scott Fray

Bear & Company
Rochester, Vermont

Bear & Company
One Park Street
Rochester, Vermont 05767
www.InnerTraditions.com

Bear & Company is a division of Inner Traditions International

Note to the reader: This book is intended as an informational guide. The remedies, approaches, and techniques described herein are meant to supplement, and not to be a substitute for, professional medical care or treatment. They should not be used to treat a serious ailment without prior consultation with a qualified health care professional.

Library of Congress Cataloging-in-Publication Data

Scully, Nicki, 1943-
  Alchemical healing : a guide to spiritual, physical, and transformational medicine / Nicki Scully.
    p. cm.
Includes index.
  ISBN 978-1-59143-015-5
  1. Healing—Miscellanea. 2. Spiritual healing—Miscellanea. 3. Occultism. I. Title.

  BF1999.S369 2003
  299'.93—dc21

                              2003010445

Printed and bound in the United States at Lake Book

10 9 8 7 6 5

Text design and layout by Virginia Scott Bowman
This book was typeset in Sabon with Civet as the display typeface

★ ☽ ★

For my beloved husband, Mark Hallert, who shares with me a magical partnership that is forever in service to the healing of our blessed Mother Earth, and All Our Relations.

CONTENTS

ACKNOWLEDGMENTS

Into my alchemical vessel I set my intention to create this book, and the various ingredients began to reveal themselves. Many people provided contributions without which this book would never have been completed, and for which I am deeply grateful.

The special influence and knowledge of a number of teachers were initially poured into my sacred cauldron: among them were Nadia Eagles, Martin High Bear, Oh Shinnah, Bethel Phaigh, and Rolling Thunder. The *prima materia* was retrieved with the help of Brian O'Dea.

Eye of newt and toe of dragon were provided by many teachers and seers extraordinaire, including Roland Barker, Gloria Taylor Brown, Bo Clark, Dr. Christine Fehling-Joss, David Groode, Charla Hermann, Christine Payne Towler, Mira Sophia, Chris Tice, Kay Cordell Whitaker, Imani White, and Reuben Wolff.

As I continued to stir the cauldron, other magi helped me hold the container as other ingredients were added. These include the entire Thoth Lineage, with special support and input from Anita Bermont, Kalita Todd Contasino, Gayle Clayton, Danielle Hoffman, Liisa Korpella, Bambi Merryweather, Joan Porter, Kathryn Ravenwood, and Laura Strobel.

When the moon waxed full and the stars aligned, the editorial input of Tina Rosa and Christine Coulter helped the mixture to coalesce. The great wordsmith, Normandi Ellis, then tasted the brew;

she shared her arcane knowledge and helped me to craft the body of the text.

A number of people sampled the first essence, and their contributions helped to purify and refine the distillation, and pushed me to make it better: Jay Moore, Ben Emmons, Elizabeth Hallert, Dennis William Hauck, Gary Leikas, Sharon Sinclair, Friedemann Schaub, M.D., Ph.D. and others who are previously mentioned.

Color and spice were added with the illustrations of Scott Fray, and the beautiful cover painting of Isis by Willow Arlenea.

No work of alchemy is complete without the infusion of Spirit, for which I have to thank my extensive healing team: Comfrey and all the plant medicine allies, Bear, the Crone, Cobra, Kuan Yin, Anubis, Sekhmet, Isis, Spider and all the spirit guides and helpers who have upheld Alchemical Healing and assisted in the healing work.

Two sorceresses from Inner Traditions • Bear & Co., project editor Laura Schlivek and copy editor Victoria Sant'Ambrogio, stepped up to the cauldron and with their own ladles stirred, shaped, and molded, and, as the earth shook and the black dog howled, we pulled forth this book.

My husband Mark Hallert, the true visionary in the family, touched every page with his insight.

And finally—words cannot convey my appreciation for my mentor and teacher, Thoth, the true architect of Alchemical Healing. It is my heartfelt prayer that these pages express the truth of his wisdom.

PREFACE

PURPOSE

HEALING IS BY NATURE an alchemical process. With clear intention and resolve, we can use our adverse situations to help us grow spiritually, emotionally, and even physically, which opens up a myriad of possibilities regarding how we choose to live our lives and how we relate to one another and the world.

All people have inherent healing abilities that, for the most part, are not recognized or acknowledged in our culture. Although our population has burgeoned since the industrial revolution and the advent of modern medical technology, many of the simple, effective, and free or easily affordable cures have been lost and largely forgotten. Western culture suffered a severe setback in this regard during the Inquisition, when healers were considered heretics and burned at the stake. In our rush for freedom in the New World, we assumed that the original inhabitants of this land were primitives, and in our arrogance, laid waste to thousands of years of cultural and spiritual development that had preceded us here. Regardless of our race or where we came from, most of us have been cut off from the wisdom of our ancestors for so long that we need help to remember ourselves. It is time to reclaim the power and pathways to knowledge that are buried deep within our psyches and our DNA. Within us dwell all the memories of our ancestors, and the ability to more fully comprehend new mysteries bursting forth from our unfolding universe. We are all mystics and sages waiting to remember what we've misplaced.

We are living during an unprecedented explosion of technology; now it is time to catch up with an equal explosion of spirituality. The purpose of this book is to further our awakening. In the course of remembering, we are not limited to what is in our own heads; we have access to the gestalt of the entire accumulated wisdom in the fullness of time. Part of the work of Alchemical Healing is to reawaken ourselves to these possibilities so that we may gain effective skill in healing. The other part is to actually transform ourselves to higher levels of awareness and ability so that we become fully healthy and accountable beings. Alchemical Healing is both a school of knowledge and a spiritual path to an enlightened state of presence.

It is important for readers of this book to know at the outset that this is primarily a hands-on manual that provides a series of initiatory steps toward mastering a powerful healing form. Alchemical Healing is a modern alchemical tradition based in the same eternal source of intelligence that sustained the high civilization of ancient Egypt and many of the great magical and alchemical traditions that still survive today.

The challenge I face in writing this book is to provide the basics, the palette and tools for the work, without limiting the creative expression of what is more an art form than a doctrine. The power of Alchemical Healing comes from the intention of its practitioners and from their willingness to suspend any personal agenda in the healing work in order to allow something new to happen each time. It requires attention, focused concentration and presence, and expanded awareness that honors intelligence and invites inspiration and assistance from the realms of spirit. Skill can be developed through practice, and by learning about the elements used, much as an artist learns about the properties of her chosen medium. True magic, however, cannot be contrived. It is the gift of grace and the Mystery.

It is, therefore, my intention to use these pages to convey as much as I can about the medium of Alchemical Healing. I will stress the importance of fostering confidence in your intuition, making relationships with the elements and allies that support the work, and learning to work with the tools and techniques I have found most useful. It is also my intention to honor those who have supported the growth of Alchemical Healing, the teachers who have been trained by me and who know the initiations and attunements at a deeper level than presented here. This is a primer; it is not a teacher's manual. Please do not take it upon yourself to teach this work to others without the extensive training required. Alchemical Healing teachers can assist you in reaching more refined levels of work, and can also share advanced techniques that are beyond the scope of this book. Whether you use this book alone, in a circle of friends or a study group, or have access to an authorized Alchemical Healing instructor,* this handbook will provide you with a vast array of innovative tools for your medicine bag.

I hope you will discover that healing as an intentional activity is a natural result of expanding your consciousness to a much broader experience of reality, one that includes the regeneration of wisdom, and one that ultimately leads to becoming a fully present, awake, and more enlightened human being.

The introductory remarks that follow in the first four chapters create a context within which the reader can identify the source and container for Alchemical Healing as a form. At the same time, they tell some relevant parts of my own life story and describe the path by which I came to discover the healing abilities that I believe are inherent in each of us. The actual hands-on work begins with Part II.

---

*For access to training programs with authorized teachers of Alchemical Healing, see Appendix II at the back of the book.

PART I

INTRODUCING
ALCHEMICAL
HEALING

1
RITE OF PASSAGE

THE CROWD WAS EXCITED. I could hear the swelling sound of thousands of fans undulating through the old building into the dressing room where I was being outfitted, growing louder and louder. It was a few minutes before midnight, December 31, 1983. I looked in the mirror and adjusted the fresh wreath of bloodred roses on my head. The grotesque makeup and diapers were weird, but the rest of my costume was comfortable—black leotard and tights painted front and back with the bones of a skeleton. A white satin banner with the number *1984* was draped across my front like a Mexican bandito's bullets, or a beauty pageant queen's sash.

The Grateful Dead always rang in the New Year with great fanfare. To the audience, I, along with my ex-husband Rock, in a matching costume but with an Uncle Sam top hat, would appear as we had for the previous five years. We were symbols of the Dead, grateful to be alive, dancing.

I could feel the excitement of the crowd mounting as I went from the dressing room to the stage and listened for the count down . . . four, three, two, one—then the huge roar from the audience as the first bars of the music erupted into a festive and rousing rendition of "Sugar Magnolia," and thousands of balloons dropped from the cavernous ceiling of the San Francisco Civic Auditorium. Rock and

I danced in the New Year tossing roses to the crowd while the great rock and roll impresario, Bill Graham, dressed as Father Time, stood atop a huge mock-up of the Earth while it rolled from the back of the auditorium all the way down to the stage. The joyfully frenzied crowd went proverbially wild.

I was still rushing with excitement and bliss as I came off the stage when a hand grabbed my shoulder and spun me around. "Come quickly!" my friend Shane cried urgently. "My sister . . ." I couldn't hear much over the music and the clamor of the crowd. He pulled me a short distance through the throng to where his sister lay, surrounded by concerned, protective people waiting for help to appear. The medics arrived at the same time as I did, and worked swiftly yet carefully to get her onto a scoop stretcher. I followed them to the place where Rock Med was set up, still not sure what had happened, and took a position at her head. I made eye contact and began pouring energy in through her crown.

The doctor was serious, all business in his demeanor, although he wore glitter on his face. He told everyone who wasn't a necessary part of his team to leave; then he looked at me and asked, "What are you doing?"

"I'm a hands-on healer," I replied. My hands were visibly vibrating as I stood there holding both hands above her without being invasive.

"Okay, stay where you are."

He then began a careful examination and quickly determined that she needed to be taken to the hospital. I learned that an overzealous fan had either jumped or fallen from the balcony and landed on Anne, then run off through the crowd. The doctor was concerned that her back might be broken. Again he turned to me.

"Will you go with her in the ambulance?"

I experienced a flood of mixed emotions. "That's up to her," I said; but when I looked back down at the frightened young face I knew I would stay with her as long as I could—and I did. We locked eyes and I kept the energy running as the ambulance sped through the streets of San Francisco, sirens blaring. It was a surreal ride. No words were shared, yet there was a deep intimacy in our connection. I felt as though my eyes were the shock absorbers that carried her through each bump and jolt on the journey. Across the gulf between her pain and my presence, I made my passage from apprentice to healer. In those defining moments, I knew fully, perhaps for the first time, who I was.

Things were even stranger at San Francisco General. Apparently New Year's Eve is a popular night at this huge hospital. There were gurneys carrying people in various levels of emergency literally littering the halls. I kept to my vigil, holding eye contact as much of the time as I could, and kept the energy flowing.

Finally it was time for Anne to enter a door through which I could not pass; yet it would be hours, even days, before her eyes did not appear in front of mine. When the door closed behind her, I turned and started down the hall—the grim reaper in roses, barefoot, passing one gurney after another occupied by the victims of revelry gone awry.

Hitchhiking wasn't as hard as I thought it would be for a chilly, barefoot skeleton. Because the hospital was overwhelmed and only admitting the most urgent of cases, in the parking lot I easily caught a ride from a van that was carrying an accident victim looking for another hospital for treatment. The driver dropped me off at the concert just at the moment when the last strains of the encore wafted out to the street, followed by the appreciative roar of the crowd.

The passage was complete. The reflection continued.

★ ☽ ★

I did not have a working knowledge of alchemy at the time I had this experience. Only in retrospect am I able to view my life with recognition of the initiations, rites of passage, and stages of the alchemical process each experience represents. What made that New Year's Eve a defining moment in my life was the realization that my commitment as a healer surpassed all other priorities. I was forty years old, and I had found myself and — with absolute certainty—my reason for being. Never again would I ask the question, What am I doing here? From this moment forward, the question would be, simply, How can I do it better? How can I accomplish more?

Alchemically, I was at both the end and the beginning. I had completed a full round of the *Opus,* the alchemical process that we continuously cycle through as we move through the stages of development in our lives. My essential nature was revealed to me. Although there is no end to becoming, the propulsive energies for the next phase of my life were set into motion.*

---

*For her part, Anne did indeed have a broken back and remained hospitalized for some time. She contacted me later to let me know how important our initial contact had been and how our energetic connection had helped her to withstand her ordeal.

2
ALCHEMY

ALCHEMY IS THE PROCESS by which each of us moves from our primal state of unconsciousness, through the various alchemical stages represented by our most elemental experiences, to the realization of full awakening, or enlightenment. It is the interactive dance through which we are constantly weaving spirit and matter into the multidimensional tapestry of life. Alchemy is a process that spirals from cycle to cycle, ever upward and forward, repeating itself as required to transform and change us through the experiences of our body, soul, psyche, and spirit. In alchemical terminology it is called the *Opus,* or *Great Work*. The higher state of consciousness and self-understanding that results includes recognition of our connection to the spirit world and awareness of the interconnectedness of all beings.

The goal of the Great Work is called, among other things, the philosophers' stone, the universal medicine, alchemical gold, and the elixir of life. It is the interpenetration of spirit and matter—the spiritualization of our material selves, and the materialization of our spiritual essence.

Alchemy has much in common with shamanism. A shaman is a multidimensional traveler who journeys into various realms of spirit to bring back power and healing for the benefit of his or her community. A shaman's development requires a breakdown of ego, and toward this end there are rites of passage that often lead to the edge of or beyond the physical, mental, and emotional tolerance of most people. I've never heard of a shaman who has not undergone ordeals that tested his mettle and stretched the envelope of his abilities. All shamans go through a process of decomposition and re-membering in order to find their personal power and abilities, and all have allies from the spirit world with whom they consult and often merge. These allies include plants, animals, minerals, elementals, and often the spirits of places. Even the realms beyond death are open to certain shamans.

As in alchemy, a shaman's body and psyche are his laboratory, and through his initiatory experiences he develops the power, the humility, and the relationships he needs to function as intercessor for others. He is also a medicine maker, often creating his cures as a result of divine inspiration.

The roots of classical alchemy are found in the Arabic, *Al Khemit,* which translates roughly as "of the black land." *Khem* is the ancient Egyptian word for Egypt herself—the land of black, fertile silt that was left after the inundation swept through the Nile Valley each year, the place of the fecund earth which, when blessed by the regenerative forces of nature, brought forth new life that grew and nourished the people.

The word *alchemy* commonly refers to a legendary medieval art by which an adept could turn lead into gold. This is only one aspect of alchemy. Those "puffers," so called because of their frantic use of the bellows, whose sole purpose was the generation of riches, were an embarrassment to true alchemists, and have maligned the reputation of an art with a much more noble objective.

For those actually engaged in the Great Work, the transmutation of metals was an allegory veiling their true goal. This goal was a superior and interior achievement—the alchemical gold of enlightenment—through which one transcends duality and illusion and becomes one with the fabric of creation, where creator and creation are one.

What is the matter? Integrated into our language is this common question, which goes for the underlying source of *that which is in need of transformation.* Some ancient texts say that the goal of the Work can only be achieved by starting with that which contains at its source some of the basic ingredient of the desired result. This ingredient is the *prima materia,* or prime matter. In Egypt, the obvious analogy was the fertile black soil itself. For the later alchemist, it is variously the base metals and/or the unconscious mind. In plant alchemy, it is the active curative essence that is rendered from the physical plant. Ultimately, alchemy is an enigma that offers seemingly paradoxical, often contradictory ground rules for a mysterious, although not insurmountable, challenge, to know ourselves fully, inside and out.

The ancient art of alchemy is easily understood by an example found in nature, the transformation that occurs over time in the creation of a diamond. The matter starts as carbon, deep within the earth. Through elemental interaction and when the appropriate amount of heat and pressure is applied and sustained, transmutation occurs—the soft black material becomes the exquisite, clear, hard, brilliant diamond.

Pressure is a fundamental part of that process, and as we explore the process of alchemy in our own lives, we discover that it is through the management of pressure that we achieve personal mastery. It is not so much about what comes to us in our life experience, but rather how we respond to it that indicates our level of mastery. Alchemically, we can see every adverse condition as a valuable part of the process, grist for the inner mill in which transmutation takes place. In healing, it is the disease that forces us to learn how to transform in order to heal.

The basic tenets of alchemy are distilled in the Emerald Tablet, one of the most quoted and studied of the guiding treatises of alchemical lore. The Emerald Tablet is attributed to Hermes Trismegistus, the legendary author of works on theosophy, magic, wisdom, and alchemy, who is associated with the Greek god

Hermes, and the ancient Egyptian god of wisdom, Thoth. The Tablet suggests that "that which is above is the same as that which is below: All that exists is of One Mind, or of One Thing, and they are the same."* It is the goal of the alchemist to bring spirit and matter into alignment and harmony. Within that relationship rests the secret of creation, and with it our ability to co-create our own reality and to heal ourselves and others.

The language used to convey ancient and medieval alchemy was purposely misleading, encoded in terms so difficult to understand that the majority of those who tried to decipher it were either led astray or forced to give up. Medieval scholars often found it to be "gibberish," a word they coined to refer to the work of Geber, an ancient Arabian alchemist whose writings they could not understand. The Great Work of alchemy was disguised in symbolic language that described the process for transmutation of the black earth of potential into the alchemical gold of illumination. In other words, alchemy described the transformation of the chaos of the mind into realization of the true essence of being.

It is important to note that I developed Alchemical Healing as a form before I undertook any formal study of classical alchemy. It has been a source of tremendous validation for me to discover the depth and breadth of the parallels between Alchemical Healing and what I now know to be true and pure alchemy. Traditional alchemy can be studied superficially; however, only direct, fresh experience brings it to life. The steps required to create the resulting elixir or stone relate directly to the experiences required to achieve mastery and enlightenment. Each stage represents an archetypal experience through which one is forced to grow in a certain way.

---

*My favorite modern translation and interpretation of the Emerald Tablet, the hermetic text that is most commonly recognized as the Rosetta stone for classical alchemists, has been written by Dennis William Hauck. His book *The Emerald Tablet: Alchemy for Personal Transformation* (New York: Penguin Compass, 1999) explores the text in detail. See Appendix I for his translation of this ancient text.

THE STAGES OF ALCHEMY

The number of operations in the alchemical process vary according to the source. Although I have seen them expressed many ways, most of the books I have consulted suggest that there are seven operations in the Great Work. These are *calcination, dissolution, separation, conjunction, fermentation, distillation,* and *coagulation.* Although there is a generally regarded succession, these operations can occur simultaneously or in a different order. Like the ancient alchemical symbol of the orobouris—the snake swallowing its tail— the steps continue to repeat themselves in the infinite cycle of birth, life, death, and rebirth. The interpenetration of these opposites—the spiritual and the corporeal—within ourselves leads to the clarity of consciousness that results in the illumined stone. It is within the body and mind of the aspirant that these processes occur. We are the alchemical vessel within which transmutation happens.

In the first stages of the work, the corporeal elements themselves, Fire, Water, Air, and Earth, work their magic on the body and/or soul. *Calcination,* the first operation, is like the fire that burns away all but what remains of substance, the ash. Most of us have experienced moments when life as we know it disintegrates. The plug is

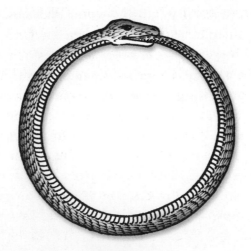

Figure 2.1.
The Orobouris

pulled, and all the systems on which we would normally rely crash, leaving us desperately adrift, in search of something to cling to that is absolutely solid and true.

Dissolution, the second operation, works to dissolve the more spiritual or psychic elements, on consciousness itself. *Dissolution* is the "solve" in *solve et coagula,* the melting of the ego that encourages the ultimate transmutation from ego to essence.

All of the processes of alchemy repeat themselves in the course of our lives, and the first two often happen simultaneously. As I reflect on the experiences in my own life, from the newly gained perspective of classical alchemy, one of the clearest calcination and dissolution operations started when I was diagnosed with cancer, just after my first book was published in 1991. I had just completed a full round of the Opus, and life was fuller and more exciting than ever. My world seemed in perfect order, and I was at the top of my game. In that singular moment when the words "you have cancer" were spoken, the world as I knew it crumbled around me, and I knew I was in for a very different future than the one I had planned.

The processes of calcination and dissolution continued through most of my chemotherapy treatment. While I lay steeping in the poisonous chemicals during an intensive four-month protocol, it wasn't just the cancer cells that dissolved. My entire understanding of myself, my judgments, and all the habits I had developed in order to survive also dissolved. I had to die to my old self, and in doing so I discovered that much of the old artificial persona was not worth resurrecting.

During the process of *separation,* the essence begins to emerge, separated out of what remains from the first two operations. From the Emerald Tablet, "The Wind carries it in its belly." Wind, and the element Air, is associated with discrimination. That which is subtle is separated from that which is gross "gently, and with great ingenuity." We are forced to develop new ways of perceiving reality in order to function. The Sufi poet Rumi, in a translation by Coleman Barks, speaks on separation: "We know separation so well because we've tasted the union. The reed flute makes music because it has already experienced changing mud and rain and light into sugarcane. Longing becomes more poignant if in the distance you can't tell whether your friend is going away or coming back. The pushing away pulls you in."

Following the calcination and dissolution that my cancer treatment provided, I was able to consciously discriminate between what were unhealthy habit patterns from my past that had contributed to my disease, and what I knew would work better for me in the future.

The hypervigilance catalyzed by the potentially fatal experience of cancer had an unexpected and beneficial side effect: I learned that with expanded awareness one can consciously hold opposites within oneself. Such ability and the resulting space it creates are hallmarks of having reached the separation stage, and a prelude to something new occurring.

The fourth operation is the *conjunction*. This joining of opposites moves one beyond duality and into a higher state, evidenced by a new perspective. As we merge our soul and our spirit, male and female, above and below, intuition and logic within our being, we become balanced and whole. It is having a foot in both worlds—like appreciating the passion and magic of sex while at the same time understanding its mechanics and chemistry.

There are *lesser* and *greater* conjunctions. If the first three operations are incomplete, or the result is still impure, a lesser conjunction occurs. Psychologically that happens when the ego refuses to die. The offspring of this conjunction is necessarily weak or deformed, and mortification, a form of death, follows. This sets off the putrefaction process and the naturally ensuing fermentation. The rotting decomposition gives way to new life as the action of digestion breeds energy.

I live in Oregon, where the winters are wet and cold and where most of the garden dies off at the end of the growing season. It is during this fallow time that the hidden work happens. The worms and bacteria in the soil eat the roots and the manure that we add and bring new life and new energy to what appeared to be dead. We see that same thing in our lives in the dark and quiet times when we are gestating new ideas and incubating inspiration.

We all have experienced lesser conjunctions where the result is not immediately sustained. It is through a kind of death and renewal that we find great benefit from what initially appear to be our most challenging situations. Bad marriages can be like that, for it is often in the reflective time after the death of a relationship that new possibilities awaken.

Cancer was certainly a case in point for me—it was during the darkest, most miserable descent into a vision quest by poisoning that I experienced the following epiphany, one of several that happened during my treatment, and one that I recognize as a pivotal healing moment.

Four close friends who had studied healing with me for many years were working on me, as they did every Monday and Tuesday evening during my weekly intensive chemotherapy protocol. They practiced the healing work we had learned during the previous ten years. We played what we intuited as appropriate music, and this evening, the music was particularly effective as a vehicle. As my friends worked the healing energies, I found myself traveling inward, deeper and deeper, until I entered a level where I recognized what felt like the patterning of genes. Several days prior, I had seen a TV show that mentioned the possibility of a damaged gene found in women with a proclivity to breast cancer. With the support of the music, the spirits, and my friends, I was able to enter deeply into my body, connect to this gene, and bring it forth, almost as though I was holding it in my hands. At that point I was left with a dilemma: I have never thought of violence as an appropriate means for making anything better. Yet here I was, my body a battlefield, armed with an arsenal of chemicals developed to deal cancer its death blows, hoping to do so without doing irrevocable damage to healthy organs and tissues. In prior sessions I'd spent a lot of time dealing with high levels of toxins and clearing them out of my systems. This time, with the magic of the moment and the intention that was being focused, I was able to direct my full attention on the gene and know it transformed and healed through love. A basic pattern in the blueprint of my being shifted from life destroying to life affirming. I felt it. I knew it.

When the music next shifted I found myself desiring to strengthen and protect my organs, particularly my heart. It was as if all of the diverse traditions of my experience blended with the eclectic qualities in the music, the hands of my friends, and all events that had contributed to the current moment—and I prayed for my heart to be opened. Layer upon layer of bright patterned veils opened to reveal yet deeper patterns until all barriers dissolved, and in that moment, the music passed through my whole unobstructed being in rushes as wind passing through a reed. I knew myself to be in total unity with all of life and all of spirit.

I felt the healing. I knew myself to be healed.

Throughout all the processes of alchemy, it is important to remember the teaching from the Emerald Tablet: "That which is Below corresponds with that which is Above, and that which is Above corresponds with that which is Below." What happens in the spirit world is a reflection of what happens in the physical world. In healing, it is easier to make the changes in the energetic or spirit world. According to the "as above, so below" tenet, those changes are reflected back into the physical body, and healing happens according to natural law.

Although the greater conjunction leads directly to the goal of the Opus, it usually requires further purification through fermentation and distillation in order to coagulate into the "stone" and achieve a complete union with the divine. The newly awakened and divinely inspired offspring is further purified through *distillation,* during which the vaporous quintessence is rendered from the new material and reintroduced as spirit in form. During this process we can observe the transmutation as it occurs, perceiving the changes with our heightened sensitivities. In distillation, we find a key mystical process by which gross elements become more rarified and closer to the divine quintessence that is the goal of alchemy. It is through an analogous process of purification that we find ourselves closer to our own divine spiritual nature.

Despite the powerful healing I had experienced, I was determined to complete my prescribed protocol. During the subsequent and final weeks of treatment, profound opportunities for magic entered and nourished my healing process. My spirit guides and allies were always with me as I continued to steep in the active processes of fermentation and distillation. Upon completion of sixteen weeks of intensive chemotherapy, with the catheter still implanted in my chest, I flew to Santa Barbara and went into the studio to produce one of my most powerful audiocassettes, *Awakening the Cobra.** During the guided journey on the tape, Cobra clears the energy channels of the listener, opens and invigorates all the chakras, and awakens the kundalini energy in the body. All seven steps of alchemy are addressed within the journey of the cobra, who is now accessible as an internal ally. Perhaps this tape was the physical expression, the living symbol of the final stage, *coagulation,* in this round of the alchemical process. The cobra had been a potent ally throughout my treatment, and I had now sufficiently comprehended her spirit so that she could extend her power through the tape and out into the world, to continue the work we had begun together.

It is in the final operation of the Great Work that the alchemist achieves his or her divine potential. Coagulation reveals pure wisdom, the incorruptible balm that heals all and transcends all aspects of the mundane world. This is the elixir of life, the philosopher's stone or universal medicine, alchemical gold.

Yet there is no end to our becoming. No sooner do we complete one round on the alchemical spiral of consciousness than we start over again. The Work is never complete. No sooner was I finished with chemotherapy and subsequent radiation treatment than I was back on the road, teaching and traveling to Egypt, and noticing how the matter had changed.

---

*The guided journey on this cassette came from the Cobra Journey in *Power Animal Meditations.*

Alchemy utilizes the four gross elements—Earth, Water, Fire, and Air—as well as the quintessential Essence that is the result of the perfected mix of these elements. Alchemy in its truest sense is the mixing of elements to create transformation. Some consider it to be the precursor to modern chemistry, Jungian and transpersonal psychology, and the Western traditions of magical arts, such as Tarot and Cabala. The same could be said of all modern healing forms that bring together these same elements in a variety of ways to assist in healing.

Alchemy relies heavily on symbolism to convey meaning, and the symbols develop their own life over time. The symbols used by the ancient alchemists, accessible in the collective unconscious of their ancestors, remain imbedded still in the collective unconsciousness of their descendants. Because of consistencies in the art and metaphysical laws of the various traditions, practitioners bring these symbols to life through the practice of modern alchemy. I have tried to clearly explain most of the symbolic language when it appears throughout this book, and you will recognize many of the symbols as integral parts of the visualizations we will use to guide us through the journey into mastery of Alchemical Healing.

As we have seen in the seven stages of alchemy, the infusion of spirit is key to the transmutation process in the more advanced operations of the Work. Spiritual inspiration is half of the equation; without it, the possibilities for genuine healing are greatly reduced. It is the co-creative nature of the relationship between ourselves and spirit that is the foundation of this path. Relationships with spirit guides provide a vital link between the spirit world and this material plane. It is similar to weaving: if the weft is spirit and the warp is matter, then where they intersect, new patterns are established. When you bring the separate elements of color, texture, line, form, skill, and intelligence together to create a preconceived design, the result of the weaving is transformation. Alchemical Healing is a practical process joining that which is above (weft) with that which is below (warp), simultaneously strengthening and healing while aligning the inner and outer realities of all that are involved.

3
THE TREASURE HUNT

THERE IS A SMALL LIVING TRADITION in Tibet known as the Terma tradition, whose purpose is to find and translate hidden treasures left by the ancient sage Padmasambava. Known as the father of Tibetan Buddhism, Padmasambava brought the Buddhist teachings from India to Tibet around fourteen hundred years ago. He was a man of great power and magic. Before he left the earth plane, he hid these treasures so that they would be found at certain times and in certain places, and by quite specific people. It is the purpose of the tertons, the adherents of this tradition, to find these termas, then translate them and bring the knowledge that they hold out into the world.

The treasures usually come in two forms: earth termas and mind termas. An earth terma is a physical manifestation such as a scroll or written teaching, or a statue, implement, or stone, that is revealed, often at great peril for the terton, whose life might depend upon being in exactly the right place at the right time. A mind terma is a complex, sophisticated thought form that coalesces in the consciousness of the terton when all preparations have been properly made and guidance is followed. Some tertons are said to return lifetime after lifetime to search out these jewels of wisdom, the time capsules of Padmasambava.*

FINDING THE PATH

My own life has been a magnificent treasure hunt, a sacred journey of Alchemical Healing, although I wasn't aware of its greater purpose during the earlier stages of the trip. I've moved from clue to clue, searching my experience for glints of brilliance, tinges of magic, the wonders of impossibility. Each clue has been a treasure in its own rite, with special intrinsic value, and each has helped me to establish my direction.

I had no concept of spirituality while growing up. Consequently, I did not always have conscious spiritual relationships. I've often wondered if there is any precedence in my family heritage for who and what I have become. I came from an ordinary family, or so it seemed to me. No stories of life in the "old country" have survived. My grandparents on both sides escaped the anti-Semitic pogroms in Russia and Lithuania near the turn of the century, and by the time I was born in New York, my parents had done their best to assimilate into mainstream American culture. When I was three, we moved out west by train to a stucco and stone house in a predominantly Jewish neighborhood of Los Angeles, just off Fairfax Avenue. When I was eight we moved to Beverly Hills, where I was raised cloistered in the illusion of my parents' social status and monetary security, both of which collapsed just before my senior year in high school when my gambler father lost his entire fortune. Reviewing that time in our lives from an alchemical perspective, I can see why alchemy is considered risky business. My father never recovered from this calcination, the most humbling experience of his life. Yet many of my enduring values were rendered from that dark time when everything that was not genuine simply vanished.

---

*Paraphrased from Tulku Thondup, *The Hidden Teachings of Tibet: An Explanation of the Terma and Traditions of Tibetan Buddhism* (Boston: Wisdom Publications, 1997).

Still, there were no indications that I would follow a healing path and become a spiritual teacher. I experienced no precognition, no strange déjà vu, no psychic phenomena. Nor did I show any special gifts or talent for healing, although as a child I loved to play doctor and brought home every broken-winged bird and malnourished stray cat I encountered.

As a matter of fact, when it comes to healing, I don't think I have any inherent gifts or am any different than anyone else. And although I always fancied myself a seeker, I was pushing forty by the time I had an inkling of my purpose in life. Only now, looking back, can I see that all relationships and events large and small conspired to lead me to the path of service to which my life is now consciously dedicated.

The shamanic path often includes the use of sacraments. When I was first introduced to LSD I did not recognize it as a sacrament, nor did I see it as a step on a shamanic path. I had dutifully followed the course my parents had charted for me, but it simply wasn't working. By my junior year in university, I had lost interest in academics and was ready to make it or break it in a world that was actually quite friendly compared to today's standards. New York held allure, so there I went, seeking to find a man to fulfill the only ambition I knew of: that of finding a husband who would support me and a social scene in which I could become my mother. Although I found a job with great potential, I was still struggling with the values of my upbringing, and I quickly grew bored. Depth and the profundity of life's adventures had not yet been made known to me.

A cousin visiting from Miami introduced me to a "longhair" who extolled the virtues of LSD. Fascinated, but skeptical, I read everything that I could find on the subject at the time. My investigations gave me the reassurance that widespread research into psychedelics had been undertaken on college campuses and in legitimate research centers. LSD was still legal, and so appeared to be much more interesting than my mundane job. I felt different from my friends and coworkers, and that sense of incongruity made me ripe for the new "hippie" movement that was still in its infancy. I returned to Los Angeles, enrolled for a short time in art school, and actively sought to transform my world according to my limited research into consciousness and psychedelics.

Thus I naively stumbled into the most pivotal moment in my life, which also was the entrance into the first serious round of the alchemical process. After opening the "doors of perception" my life changed radically. I immersed myself in the experience, if not the culture, of LSD. My day job at that time was as secretary to the comptroller of Four Star Television. At night I observed the goings-on of the hippies on Sunset Boulevard from a safe distance, and on weekends I explored my expanding consciousness with LSD. Because there were no laws against psychedelics at that time, I had no fear of reprisals. In my innocence I reveled in a remarkable, storybook experience of color and insight, vision and joy. I dove into my psyche and my sexuality, released from the confines of my upbringing. Although I thoroughly enjoyed being a kid with the run of the candy store, awareness of the spiritual magic didn't come until much later, perhaps partially because of my secular background, but also because I had no spiritual elders or role models. Even so, my direction was changing, and as I embraced the internal fires of calcination and the simultaneous dissolution of the only road map I had, the doors of my old life closed one by one and I was forced to move to the next level of the unknown.

At the end of 1966 I quit my job and moved from Los Angeles to San Francisco. My conviction that I could remain unchanged by the hippie movement evaporated the moment I moved into the red, yellow, and blue Victorian time warp of a house on the corner of Sutter and Lyon streets. There I discovered the world of psychedelic community, drug dealing, and rock-and-roll. My experience, however, was not all happiness and bliss. While the flower children were dancing in the streets of San Francisco, I was again experiencing several operations in my personal alchemical process—calcination, dissolution, separation, and most certainly, the mortification aspect of fermentation. I became embroiled in a terrifying marriage that, in retrospect, I see as the tempering of the steel of my being.

My first husband was a notorious drug smuggler whose main talent was to invoke fear—in friends and enemies alike. I first allowed him to become my lover during a vulnerable, high-dosage psychedelic moment. I had not yet learned the humility and respect required of psychedelic research. I was ill prepared mentally and emotionally for such explorations, and the results were catastrophic.

Goldfinger, as he was infamously known in the Haight-Ashbury district, was born Ken Connell—a fiery red-haired wild man, mostly of Irish descent. Sharp-minded and ruthless, he sheltered a tender soul within the huge barrier he had built to separate himself from his military parents, who were for some time alcoholics who blamed him for the death of his older brother during a childhood accident.

While I was completely open and vulnerable, he gladly accepted credit for the magical experience I was having, and I was willing to give it to him. My attempts to sustain the levels of love encountered in the altered space of our primary conjunction proved impossible. The resulting schism in my psyche grew during the early months of our relationship, until my mind, weakened from the combination of abuse, chemicals, and living a lie, could no longer take the dichotomy and I lost all perspective. During a particularly potent mescaline and LSD trip I followed a storm tunnel in my mind and ended up frozen with terror, in a semicatatonic state. I could not speak and experienced extreme paranoia, during which I believed the TV and radio were talking to me. I lost more than my ego that day and in the weeks that followed. Unable to deal with my interpretations of the haranguing voices, I attempted suicide three times, finally waking up from a two-and-a-half-day coma in the hospital. Caught climbing out the window, I was strapped down on a gurney and taken to a mental hospital. When I was released some weeks later, Ken convinced me that I could not survive without his help, and that he needed marital control to make sure nothing bad happened to me.

Our wedding was held at the Straight Theater in Haight-Ashbury late that summer. It was a classic hippie wedding. I wore a 1930s satin wedding gown; most of the guests were in costume. Janice

Joplin sang, and her band, Big Brother and the Holding Company, made the music.

In that marriage, I was cloistered from both the conventional world and the evolving consciousness of the hippies. But in the Woodstock summer of 1969, I finally emerged, pregnant with my first daughter, Spirit Acacia. Concern for the welfare of my coming child had given me the strength to make and sustain a complete break with her father.

I was six weeks pregnant when I fell in love with Rock Scully. He was a manager of the psychedelic rock band, the Grateful Dead, for the first twenty years of their stellar career. I told him I was pregnant. "You will be so beautiful," he replied, totally sincere. I was smitten.

I followed the band to the famous festival at Woodstock where Rock and I frolicked in the rain, swam in the lake, and fell more deeply in love. Over the next few years, he not only gave me sanctuary, but also provided me with the opportunity to heal myself and become part of the leading edge of a musical/spiritual lifestyle that shaped my character and paved the way for me to become a healer.

I was determined to be the best mother I could be; but my lifestyle was unstable. Spirit was barely three months old when we lost our home to fire. This new round of calcination once again stripped me of all outward semblance of a foundation and forced me to find strength and consistency within. Our family of three lived as gypsies in a pick-up truck camper shell hung with velvet tapestries for the next year or so, parking at various friends' homes, enjoying a wonderful sense of freedom. When I was pregnant again with my second daughter, Sage, we found a great place in Mill Valley. Having two children and a home to sustain became my full-time occupation, although as I gradually returned to mental strength and competence, I was able to expand my interests and my participation in our large extended family.

Sadly, our life was marred by Rock's ever-increasing drug use: he was sinking deeper and deeper into habitual use of both cocaine and opiates. I adored him, and I tried hard not to notice as he became more and more removed from us. In the spring of 1974, through a series of magical circumstances, we were given a rustic old homestead ranch in Sonoma County. It was like being thrown a lifeline, an opportunity for healing for our family.

I fell in love with the land the moment I saw it: picture postcard red clapboard buildings trimmed in white—two small houses and a barn in a private little emerald valley, filled with daffodils and a large rock-terraced garden that included a young dwarf apple orchard.

I hoped the new land would give Rock a reason to be at home. It didn't. I, on the other hand, stayed on the land and learned a lot.

I became a pioneer mom. I chopped the wood, carried the water, ground wheat into flour, baked bread in our wood cook stove, grew a garden, preserved the food, sewed the girls' dresses and Rock's shirts on an antique treadle sewing machine, and drove the kids across the county so they could attend a Waldorf school. These active years of fermentation added greatly to my sense of self, in both spiritual and material ways. I became stronger than ever before and for the first time could see myself as capable. The land gave me a base for the development of my spirituality, for it was here that I began embracing alternatives in living and healing.

At the health food store in Guerneville there was a kiosk where a beautiful gypsy-looking woman, Rosemary Gladstar, dispensed herbs and herbal knowledge. We became friends, and I would attend the weekend gatherings where she brought together teachers who shared health and spirituality teachings such as kinesiology, astrology, Tarot, and herbology. It was Rosemary who first encouraged me to learn something that I could teach, and inspired me with her unique expressions of magic and healing.

When I moved to Oregon in 1981, Rosemary moved her herb school to the land in Sonoma County. The California School of Herbal Studies continues, although under different direction. It is a fine school that is still tending the gardens and training great herbalists.

THE GRATEFUL DEAD AND SHAMANISM

I would have to say that the Grateful Dead band was a significant teacher—not the individuals in the band, but the music they created, and the culture and opportunity that galvanized around them. The value of the Grateful Dead has always been to achieve spirituality through expanded consciousness, music, joy, and celebration. Some got it on deeper levels than others.

The music was alive with a spirit of its own. We could soar on its melodies and rhythms—explore consciousness, tickle the edges of the universe, and surf the far reaches of the unknown in an intricate dance of light, sound, and color, trusting that we would be held safe in its graceful enchantment. Although I still had no idea what was in store for me, it was in these realms that I first encountered and recognized healing power.

I remember noticing light pouring off my hands one particularly psychoactive evening in the early 1970s during a concert at San Francisco's Winterland Auditorium, and attempting to direct it to where it could do some good. I knew then that this light had the power to heal, but it would take years of searching and study before I would attain the knowledge and authority needed to use it consistently. Meanwhile, emerging visions of a paradigm of harmony and respect were subtly (sometimes not so subtly) shaping my character and future.

My first introduction to Native American shamanism came in the fall of 1969. Rolling Thunder, a Cherokee medicine man, traveled to Marin County from his home in Carlin, Nevada, for the purpose of ministering to a rash of medical problems in the Grateful Dead family. I was Rolling Thunder's chauffeur for the day as we made the rounds so that he could perform healings. We stopped first at the hospital in Novato where two of our group of friends were recovering, one from a car accident and the other from liver disease.

Rolling Thunder cut an unusual figure as we entered the hospital. He was in his midfifties at the time and just revealing himself to the Western world as a medicine man and healer. Although there was nothing unusual in his manner of dress, his well-worn, western-style felt hat had an eagle feather tucked into its woven band, and he carried himself with a unique confidence. He looked at the people on whom he was working with a slight squint, as though he were seeing into two worlds.

The hospital setting formed a backdrop for an eye-opening glimpse of a method of healing quite different from the Western medical model with which I was most familiar. From among his paraphernalia Rolling Thunder brought out an abalone shell in which he placed and lit some sage leaves. He used the smoke to smudge and cleanse the room of negativity, incidentally setting off the smoke alarm. Rolling Thunder used an eagle feather like a surgical tool, although at the time my untrained eyes could not grasp the meaning of his movements; and he smoked his corncob pipe in a way that I would later understand to be sacred.

Our next stop was to be the home of the late Jerry Garcia, lead guitarist for the Grateful Dead, who was in a battle with bronchial pneumonia. On the way we bought some chicken meat. When we got to the house we built a fire in the back yard, down by the stream. Rolling Thunder smudged everyone with sage. He sprinkled corn pollen on Jerry, who was in bad shape. Things started to intensify as the medicine man began to sniff out the demon of the disease, moving right onto Jerry's body, sniffing and sensing, looking for the source of the problem. Then he began to suck. With snarling sounds he sucked the malady out of Jerry's chest. You could tell that they were doing battle, the shaman and the disease. It was like a tug of war, and with every gain he would spit into the meat. After he had completed this part of the process, he took the meat and put it in the fire. For his finale, Rolling Thunder went down to the stream and threw up.

We were all astonished by this unusual behavior. But the most remarkable thing was that Jerry was healed. Interestingly, he said that in his own way he could feel and even see the battle that was going on as Rolling Thunder was pulling the spirit of the disease out of him. When it was done, he knew that he was no longer sick, only tired from the battle.

That experience catalyzed a new direction in my life. I realized that I had been living in a kind of vacuum, and that there were many mysteries, many different, exciting possibilities that had never occurred to me. I began to pay attention to the Native American way of living on the earth, and this became my spiritual base. I learned that there were at least five hundred different languages in the multitude of unique and diverse Native American tribes. If there is a common thread that goes through all their teachings it is a respect for the spirits of Earth and an honoring of the elements of nature.

The deepest mystery, which also turned out to be the most solid foundation of my spiritual journey, slipped into my life quietly and unbidden. In May of 1974 the Grateful Dead played a concert in Missoula, Montana, where they were quietly honored by being entrusted with a sacred Pipe, known in the Lakota language as *Cannunpa* (pronounced cha•n̄ū•pa), the most sacred of tools. Standing Black Arrow, a ghost dancer and carver of the Blackfeet tribe, had been directed in a vision to make a sacred Cannunpa for the Grateful Dead. When it was completed, he invited twenty-three medicine men and women to a ceremony in which they smoked and consecrated the Cannunpa. According to my friend and first teacher, Oh Shinnah,* I was described as the future keeper. When the Grateful Dead came to Montana, Oh Shinnah and Standing Black Arrow's son delivered it to Rock, in order that it would come into my hands.

As I unpacked Rock's things when he returned, I came upon a leather bundle that I had never seen before. When I held it up it unrolled, and the pieces of a Native American Pipe fell onto the bed. I was immediately struck by its beauty and presence. Although I had no knowledge of the ways of the sacred Pipe, I felt a strong sense of reverence.

From Rock I was able to learn a bit of the Cannunpa's history and some basic rules for its use according to the instructions that

---

*Oh Shinnah is an Apache, Mohawk, and 1/8 Stot elder, living on Rainbow Mountain in Montana.

were given to him along with the Pipe. The instructions included never to smoke it with anyone using drugs or alcohol, never to use it in the presence of menstrual blood, and never to turn it counter-clockwise. I was to make prayers for the band and our extended family and fans, and for all our needs. I was told then that until the appropriate teachings came to me I was to adapt the Four Directions ceremony I had seen Rolling Thunder do many times. And, finally, that the Cannunpa would teach me. Little did I know how much!

I began to use the Cannunpa quietly, at first only with my family and close friends. The responsibility that comes with being a Pipe carrier was something that I intuited from the start, though the magnitude of it seeped into my awareness only as time and events engendered a deeper understanding of the traditions I was guided to explore.

In my quest for spiritual development and knowledge, I went in the directions indicated to me by the sacred Cannunpa and traveled deep into my own shadow, out into the reservations and lodges of the elders, and to numerous Sun Dances and other sacred traditional ceremonies. On this path I learned humility and compassion. I found a way to know my connection to the medicine wheel of life and the ancestors who prayed for us seven generations ago.

As an alchemical symbol, the Cannunpa is a true marriage of opposites. It is the union of the masculine and feminine—the receptive bowl joined with the generative stem. It is said that the whole of the universe is in harmony when the two are connected, and so it is. The eagle feather that hangs between them, like the feather of Maät to the ancient Egyptians, represents the truth, the cosmic balance and order that holds the whole of creation together. The sacred Pipe lives as a symbol of how the material and spiritual worlds intersect.

How can I emphasize the depth of importance of this sacred Way on my path? Suffice it to say that the Cannunpa has been a powerful teacher that has influenced every aspect of my life. It has given me a sense of support and validation for my presence and purpose in this life. It has been the foundation of my spiritual path and remains a mainstay of counsel in every important movement and decision.

While exploring the Red Road in search of understanding what had come to me, I encountered deep concern from my Native friends and occasional antagonism from those who did not know me regarding the exploitation of Native American spiritual ways. Many Native people still feel outrage at the numerous *wasichus,* white people, who buy, sell, and "teach" Native American spirituality, and who disrespectfully carry sacred Pipes.

I cannot pass judgment as to whether a person should follow one path or another. However, if you are called to the Cannunpa or find yourself resonating with any indigenous cultural and spiritual ways, please hold those ways sacred and with the utmost respect. It is possible for non-Native people to respectfully honor the ways that are shared with us, and there is a great deal we can learn. The Red Road is not an easy road, however, and it is not for everyone. Most importantly, it is not appropriate for us to change the ways we are shown. If you do feel called, allow this deep and spiritual magic to happen in its own time and in its own way so that you will become a responsible steward of whatever sacred knowledge is coming toward you, for the commitment it requires is not to be taken lightly. Having responsible and respectable teachers is imperative; their appearance in your life is part of the magic and the message. In the same way, running out and purchasing a sacred Pipe is not the best approach to receiving one. Do pay attention to your dreams.

★ ☽ ★

As I sought to understand why this medicine bundle came to us and what it meant to carry it, I began to shape my commitment to a life of service, using the Cannunpa to pray for clarity and direction. I learned early on that ritualizing a prayer with the Cannunpa built a basin of attraction that aligned all forces to fulfill that prayer. The more I prayed for clarity, the clearer I became with regard to my spiritual path. The more I prayed to become a servant for the healing of Mother Earth and her people, the more tools I attracted to help me to achieve that goal, and the more opportunities appeared so that I could utilize what I was learning.

The Cannunpa is still an integral part of my life and is still accessible to family and friends from that era.

The next big clue in the treasure hunt of life led me to Egypt!

EGYPT'S MYSTERY

In September of 1978 the Grateful Dead gave three concerts at the Great Pyramid in Egypt, climaxing two weeks of adventure and magic. Given free reign on the Giza Plateau, we clambered all over the pyramids, inside and out. My first "*ohm*ing" experience was in the King's Chamber, with a number of our entourage. To this day I cannot be in the presence of ohming without remembering the peculiar resonance that so startled me that first time.

At dawn each morning I would walk from the Mena House, our hotel, to the Sphinx, where the guards would let me stand between its paws and spend sunrise offering cornmeal and making prayers. Later, I would sit quietly in the "pit," a chamber deep beneath the pyramid that was neither lit nor open to the public at that time. A friend and I had convinced the guards to let us enter the narrow passageway, and, with stubs of candles (flashlights felt out of place here) we would inch our way down the deep shaft on our butts. There in the darkness we entered the uniquely expansive energy of a great, unfathomable mystery.

During the days, when we were not investigating the pyramids, our ragtag band of intrepid tripsters spilled out into the neighboring villages and engaged in magical encounters fraught with layers of spiritual meaning and synchronicity. Although most of us were ignorant of the Egyptian Mysteries at that point, we nevertheless sensed that we were responding to something big. We saw ourselves as emissaries of peace and joy, and we felt sure that our presence was both amusing and uplifting for our surprised hosts.

Early one morning in predawn darkness I began my climb to the top of the Great Pyramid with a local guide, Farad. It was steeper than I imagined. I forced myself beyond the vertigo that gripped me as I scrambled from one giant granite block to the next. By the time I reached the top, the sun was cresting the horizon, a huge globe of pale golden light, rising from the hazy city skyline, pierced by graceful minarets. A small group was already there when I arrived, hushed and reverent. Our awe never subsided, but eventually we all climbed back down together and followed my guide for quite a distance across the desert and into the village where his family lived. His wife spoke no English. She prepared breakfast for us, squatting in front of a couple of propane burners in a small, almost bare room. She dressed me in her flowing black village dress, and wrapped my head in her long black scarf. The special knot she used to hold the scarf in place conveyed to all Egyptians exactly which village the wearer came from. Farad told me to keep my distance from the others in our group, and during the long walk back along the roads of Giza, I found myself reflected in the eyes of every Egyptian woman I passed. Because of my clothing, they looked at me directly with penetrating gazes. It was during these exchanges that I first glimpsed the depths of my loving connection with Egypt.

My life was forever changed. Although I knew I would return, I could not yet know or understand the pull that would keep bringing me back to Egypt—her people, her magic, and the pervasive phenomena of synchronicity.

As the magic would have it, another gift had come to me that morning. At the top of the pyramid I met Zuni for the first time. She had traveled from the states for the concerts, and because of the auspicious moment of our meeting, we decided to become immediate friends and go into business together—traveling to Egypt.

Zuni and I returned to Egypt three weeks after leaving and twice more in 1979, supporting our travels with an import business. My attempts to understand my connection to the source of the magic during these times were modest at best. The monuments and temples of Egypt are very old and many are well preserved. Though they are the pride of a great nation, there is currently little appreciation in Egypt for the spiritual vitality that still resonates in those walls. It would be some time before the true reason for my passion for Egypt would reveal itself.

During one tour of the land of the Pharaohs, we sailed down the Nile from Luxor to Aswan on a *felucca,* an ancient type of small sailing boat, for four days. We were traveling with friends, including my daughter Acacia and Zuni's daughter Amber. We fished, bathed, and swam in the river, and slept on the deck of the boat under the stars.

One bright morning while moored on a bar in the nether zone between here and there, Amber took a dive off the edge of the boat into what she thought was deep water. It was only knee deep at most. She came up screaming, but she couldn't move because of the compression to her spine. We pulled her out of the water and laid her on the deck of the boat. We were all stunned, and helpless. I remember the next moments as if in slow motion. First was the panic when we realized that between us we had just enough skill in first aid to apply a Band-Aid to a small cut. Lacking in any training beyond the use of quartz crystals that I had received from Oh Shinnah, I grabbed the small one I'd brought with me and went to work, focusing my intention and praying for divine intervention, while holding my hands over Amber. The pain abated, and Amber was able to move soon after, fully regaining her mobility.

It was time to find a teacher or focus for my studies that would help me to accomplish the goal that had moved to the forefront of my mind—the goal of becoming a healer.

4
DISCOVERING THE
HEALER WITHIN

REIKI

By the fall of 1980 it had become apparent that my marriage was not going to survive, and that I needed to make a move in order to focus more attention on my children and my personal growth. I sought direction internally and determined to move to Eugene, Oregon, where I had a few friends and some good memories from previous visits.

It was spring of 1981, and I had just made the move when I heard about and began to study Reiki. The late Bethel Phaigh was a wonderful teacher who inspired confidence. She had a strong background in Gestalt therapy and Hawaiian Huna, and she was initiated into Reiki by Takata, the Japanese woman who had been entrusted with the Reiki lineage directly from its founder, Usui, in Japan. Takata brought Reiki to Hawaii from Japan to keep it safe during World War II.

Reiki is a powerful and simple healing tool. It gives permission to the initiate to know and direct the Universal Life Force energy for healing. I feel we have allowed certain intrinsic gifts to atrophy for lack of use, and the Reiki initiations jumpstart the process of reawakening them by making us aware of who we can be as an instrument of healing, and how easily our intention can be converted to action.

Because of our cultural prohibitions, we need permission to heal. All our lives we are told that this healing power is outside of us. It's given to doctors and ministers. "Special" beings are occasionally touched with the healing power, often after near-death ordeals or when their head hits cement at just the right angle. It's also given to mothers, whose caring hands exude the energy of love and soothe the pains of the bruises and diseases of childhood.

The tradition of laying on of hands is as old as love. It is often recognized by the most sensitive among us, many of whom are afraid to acknowledge possessing the power, for those who are "touched" often experience alienation from those around them. In indigenous cultures where such gifts are honored, lineages carry the magic in bloodlines. To some it is passed on by initiation.

Reiki is based on the premise that all humans carry an antenna that attracts the Universal Life Force existing in the ambient field of creation that surrounds us. When we raise the antenna, our intention connects the charge, and the need of the recipient draws the energy through our bodies and out of our hands. Like light filling a dark closet, the Reiki energy banishes pain and illness.

The Usui system of Reiki is very specific in its pathway to light. It utilizes mystical symbols, hidden in initiatory secrecy, to awaken the energy and open the doorways to its wonderfully direct source. And it is very effective.

I decided to take the first level of Reiki with Bethel, and my experience of the initiations was quite unremarkable. It was frustrating to be in a class with people who could feel things that simply were not evident for me. Intellectually I understood the process, based on personal experience of the energy coursing through my body at Grateful Dead concerts. Yet even with the Reiki initiations, all sensitivity to the energy escaped me when called on to experience it on demand.

The class took four evenings, with attunements at the beginning and end of each evening. Everyone participating could feel the awakening of the energy except me. By the third night I figured that I just wasn't getting it. I asked Bethel to please give me the final initiations because I wouldn't be coming the last evening.

The following day I went to Portland to meet with a friend. I proposed a Reiki session to see if I could feel the energy outside the context of class. Although he was relatively healthy, my friend's lifestyle was such that I knew a treatment on his liver would certainly be beneficial. When I placed my hands over his liver, my hands lit up as though I had just plugged them into a wall socket. The current was so strong that my friend's dogs, who had been sleeping upstairs at the far end of a very large home, came galloping downstairs to demand their fair share. It seemed as though the Reiki initiations had happened outside of time: as though the attunements took effect all at once. It was a remarkable feeling, one of palpable life force coursing from my hands into his body.

My excitement was as vibrant as the energy. I understood the gift of Reiki suddenly, as best I could at that moment, and I couldn't wait for more.

When I returned to Eugene the next day, Bethel gave me the second-level initiations and symbols and a brief description of their uses, then sent me off on my own to learn how to use them. To this day I incorporate these tools as important elements for use in my personal healing practice. Many of the students who come to me have already taken Reiki and find my practice compatible with what they've learned.

After a year or so of enthusiastically practicing Reiki at every opportunity, it became decision time. It was 1982, and at that time, if you chose to be a Reiki master, that became your life work in a very exclusive way. Although I was enthusiastic about Reiki, I never practiced it in the usual form of Reiki sessions, where you would place your hands on specific locations on the body in a certain order. I was more of an emergency room kind of practitioner. "Oh, it hurts? Let me see if I can help . . ."

At that point my close friends, Phyllis Furumoto, the lineage bearer of the Usui system of Reiki, and her husband at the time, Michael Hartley, suggested that I give some thought to taking a more shamanistic direction, because they recognized shamanic initiations in some of the experiences that I'd had in my life.

Certain powerful experiences that would be construed by some as psychotic breaks could be seen by others as shamanic initiations. My psychedelic history was rife with potent magical experiences of a shamanic nature. And my experience with the Grateful Dead also moved me into altered states and other dimensions.

Michael and Phyllis were able to put these experiences in a context that allowed me to understand them as pivotal moments in my journey of becoming a healer. As a result of this conversation, there was a subtle shift in my intention, which affected the direction of my life in ways that I could not have predicted.

HUNA

On my thirty-ninth birthday I helped cater a rock and roll concert not far from Eugene. That evening when I returned home, I found my house had been violated by burglars who obviously had knowledge of where my valuables were hidden. I was left penniless, in debt in fact, and unable to continue the renovations I had begun on my ramshackle home. With serious questions in my mind about how to proceed, I traveled to San Francisco to seek counsel from a seer who had been recommended to me. Frieda Waterhouse was a Jewish Sufi in her late seventies who practiced Huna, the sacred spiritual teachings from Hawaii. She was a tiny woman, wrinkled and wizened, sharp and clear. She started her reading with an invocation of the "Ancient of Days," the masters of Huna, whom she described briefly to me. She then told me that the robbery I had suffered would help me to remember that my security does not depend on a cache of Egyptian gold and sumptuous jewels, but rather upon my knowing the true source of all abundance.

As for the Reiki, "as wonderful and beautiful as Reiki is, for you it is but a step along the way." And she described a healing form that I could not yet conceive of: "Picture a hand outstretched but not touching . . ." She went on to describe the form that my next teacher, Nadia Dagelus (now the late Nadia Eagles), was later to teach me.

Nadia was just starting to teach Huna when I heard about her. Because of Frieda's reading, the word *Huna* rang a bell. Nadia was a brilliant, eccentric woman with a photographic memory that retained all the knowledge from the voluminous metaphysical library that consumed most of her living quarters. She could recount almost verbatim passages from obscure texts, an ability that I found both impressive and daunting. She combined the knowledge from her studies with the initiatory rites that had been taught to her and had developed a body of esoteric work that contained a huge repository of metaphysical essentials.

In the Hawaiian language, many words have multiple meanings. The word *Huna* means secret or hidden treasure. It also refers to the sacred wisdom of the Hawaiian spiritual tradition. The Kahunas are the keepers, or the priesthood, of that sacred wisdom. There are specialties in the Huna tradition that require unique training, yet the underlying principles are consistent with many of the most sophisticated modern psychological beliefs.

Very simply put, human consciousness is divided into three levels of self: High Self, Middle Self, and Low or Hidden Self. Both the High and Low Selves are shared pools of consciousness, similar to the Upper and Lower Worlds of the Australian aboriginal tribes, and the superconscious and subconscious levels in many psychological perspectives. Through our High Selves we are connected with cosmic consciousness, our ancestral wisdom spirits, and our oversouls. This higher self is called the *aumakua*, the source of our wisest guidance. The Middle Self is the *uhane*, our egoic self. It is that with which we identify as individuals. It is our Middle Self who perceives from the unique vantage point of our bodies in space and time and interprets the messages from the aumakua and from the *aku*, the

Low Self. The aku is our collective subconscious. It stores memory and is in charge of the autonomic functions of our physical body. The aku is impressed by ritual and does not distinguish between what is real and what comes in the imaginal realms of dreams, visions, or shamanic experience. That is why initiatory and shamanic journeys and guided visualizations are so powerful and effective. When the Low Self has an experience, it signals the Middle Self, and the psyche and physical body respond, regardless of the realm in which the event occurs.

Nadia taught me to heal others using the principles of Huna blended with the Western magical traditions and her studies of ancient Egypt. She taught me the importance of forgiveness, fundamental to the practice of Huna, and also the element system that is incorporated in my work. The psychic surgery procedures she shared are still viable in Alchemical Healing

Despite my difficulty with visualizations, Nadia's confidence and direction engendered considerable acceleration in my growth and transformation. I quickly became one of her favorite students, probably because I was so enthusiastic, willing to do the work, and fearless in taking the risks of applying what she taught me to real life situations. We would spend endless hours late at night on the phone, for I was by now dedicated to the treasure hunt and hungry for clues. And I like to think that my constant stream of questions pushed her to dive more deeply into her own cauldron of knowledge and intelligence.

I was the first of Nadia's students to receive transmissions and teach the first levels of her work. Transmission is an initiatory process within which knowledge and authority is passed directly from one person to another. It was now the fall of 1983. I did not feel ready to teach because there was so much I felt I still had to learn, and so much that I could not articulate nearly as well as Nadia. But I was raising my two daughters alone with limited savings, no source of income, nor any useful job experience or skills. Necessity provided the final push, and the timing was perfect. Sometimes we teach what we need to learn, and in the teaching, I gradually integrated the principles and practices that had been taught to me.

It was through the study of Huna that I came face to face with the Egyptian pantheon, with whom I have since developed a great intimacy.

MEETING MY MENTOR

Through a guided journey similar to those I will share in the course of this book, Nadia introduced me to Thoth, the mentor for my work. It was 1985 and I was receiving the transmission that would enable me to teach the advanced levels of Nadia's work. One of the many aspects of this transmission was a journey to a council that included nine members of the Egyptian pantheon. Nadia instructed me that when I went before the council, one of its members would come forward as my teacher and mentor. I felt so intimidated that when I stood before the council and Thoth stepped forward, he appeared immense; I could only see his belt buckle, yet I clearly knew it was Thoth. Thoth is the Egyptian god of wisdom who expresses an elevation of consciousness that elucidates wise choices. It took me quite some time to realize the gift of this introduction, because I was too intimidated to develop my relationship with him.

It was nearly a year later, and not long after one of my students perceived his protective presence around me, that I realized Thoth was always with me. Still later, I came to understand that he is also within me, the divine aspect of inherent wisdom to which I aspire, and from which my wisest decisions are made. He is the source of divine inspiration that infuses my life and my work. Thus began a distillation process that is only now culminated through the completion and publishing of this book.

I started paying attention. Feeling less timid, I found I was able to relate with him more directly, eye to eye. Consequently, I found him to be of immeasurable value—easily accessible, full of humor, and clearly my staunchest ally in the spirit world. As I became more confident in myself, he became my greatest source of guidance and knowledge.

Every aspect of my life and work changed when I affirmed my relationship with Thoth. The joy of the chase, of seeking and finding each step of the path, became part of an intricate game—the treasure hunt took on a new dimension in which I proceeded from clue to clue in a more conscious way. My unique body of work began to reveal itself. I asked lots of questions, and it seemed I always got more than I asked for in my search for truth and wisdom.

Everyone's creative process is different, and my relationship with my muse was no exception. Thoth's way of introducing me to the animal totems that comprise *Power Animal Meditations,* and subsequently to the practices of Alchemical Healing, was joyful, humorous, and endlessly fascinating: initially Thoth appeared with a huge vulture, obviously Egyptian in nature and style.* Vulture often appears as a totem around a person when big changes are about to happen in that person's life. She watches and waits for the right moment.

That moment came for me one evening following a day of practice with several of my students. Brian saw Thoth and the vulture as clearly as if they were in physical bodies, sharing space in the room with us. They were waiting to be noticed, and Brian had both the vision and the sensitivity to recognize their presence. Thoth instructed him to guide me, and although I was unable to "see" them visually, I felt and knew them to be present. As I followed

---

*I did some research to see who this vulture was and discovered two important Egyptian vulture deities: the goddesses Mut (pronounced *moot*) and Nekhbet. Mut is the wife of the creator god, Amun. She is one of the most ancient mother archetypes, usually portrayed as a woman wearing a vulture headdress. Nekhbet is seen on all the lintels of the temples, holding the symbol for infinity in her talons. It is she, along with the cobra goddess, Uadget, who appears on the double crown of the pharaoh. The vulture is associated with the High Self, the cobra, closer to the ground, with the Low Self, or unconscious mind. They are the guardians of Upper and Lower Egypt, which also represent the upper and lower realms of consciousness.

Brian's directions, Mut presented me with a purple-black egg, flecked with gold, and Thoth bade me to take it into my belly. What followed was the journey that is the alchemical pathway I continue to use to take people into the presence of Thoth (see page 52) and the subsequent journey with Mut to the Crone* during which the "stone," the first matter or prima materia, was initially placed within me, the beginning of the Opus. I remember being told that the stone that was being inserted was the *universal medicine,* although at the time I had no idea what it meant.

Almost immediately, within days of the initiation, the cauldron that the egg had revealed during the journey started to bubble and boil, and the beings within it began to introduce themselves. The alchemy process was happening within both my body and my consciousness; the subtle energies of spirit were separating from the chaos of the collective unconscious within. These intelligent entities would appear mostly as animal totems to my students during classes and healing sessions, and I recorded the journeys they brought. I encouraged my students to build relationships with these totemic characters, and I paid attention to how they developed. It took four years to complete the original research, and another to complete the first edition for publishing.

CANCER

Please don't get the idea that just because you have clear and wonderful guidance it will always be easy. The publishing of my first book was magically conceived and smoothly executed; but when it came time for promotion, things changed. I was fully engaged in the details of arranging my book tour and had other great plans when I discovered the lump in my right breast. My response was to check my calendar to see when it would be convenient to deal with it. It was December, and many women were trying to get their mammo-

---

*See *Power Animal Meditations* and The Cauldron of Thoth audiocassette.

grams before the insurance year ran out. I finally got an appoint-
ment and somehow had the presence to take the technician's hand
and get her to feel the lump. When the mammogram came out clean,
she called me back saying, "I felt a lump, but it didn't show up." I
went back in the next morning, and this time the news was not
good. I would have to have a biopsy. It was now almost Christmas
and I was leaving on December 28 to lead a two-week tour to Egypt.
There was no one in my town that could schedule me that fast, so I
called a surgeon who was a family friend in San Francisco. He had
me call his son, who arranged for the surgery to happen on
Christmas morning in Eureka, California, where I could stop while
driving to San Francisco from Eugene, on my way to Cairo.

Bad news. Not only was the tumor malignant, the surgeon hadn't
been able to get clean margins. "Do you still plan to go to Egypt?"
Of course. "Well, call as soon as you get home, because you don't
want to wait any longer than that."

No sooner had the stone from one alchemical round been
brought to fruition than the cycle began again. I celebrated by going
to hear the Grateful Dead, then left the next morning to take thirty-
two people through the mysteries in Egypt. It was actually perfect
timing, for where else could I get such clear and direct guidance?
Egypt was my power place. What's more, most of the participants
on that trip were healers. Dealing with cancer during this journey
forced me to participate in a deeper way than ever before, and we
all benefited. On the way home I stopped in San Francisco for a second surgery, a re-excision where the surgeon again attempted to get
clean margins and took some lymph nodes to check for metastasis.
Once again, no clean margins; and yes, a number of the nodes were
infected.

My guidance was clear: to entrust myself to the medical estab-
lishment while augmenting their choice of protocols with my own
and other alternative support. Because of the aggressiveness of my
cancer, I was given a not-yet-published experimental chemotherapy
program that laid me out for four long months, followed by two
months of radiation.

So much for my promotional tour.

Looking back, I would have to say that the gifts I received from my cancer experience were well worth the misery. I don't recommend asking for such a journey, but if it comes to you, you can regard it as an opportunity, and I suggest you honor it in that way. My bout with cancer was the crucible that held the distilling fire that refined my path, and from which I emerged a stronger and more committed healer.

Soon after my treatment concluded, Thoth showed me the next clue in the treasure hunt: a vision of the two of us silhouetted against a glowing evening sky, looking up at the stars. He told me it was time to connect to his source so that I could bring in the next level of the work. And so it continues . . .

PART II

BASIC
ALCHEMICAL
HEALING

5
INITIATION

IN MANY INDIGENOUS CULTURES powerful puberty rites provide the launching platform for the passage from youth to adulthood. These are often difficult ordeals that test the endurance of the initiate. They also ensure that the tribal and cultural mores and traditions are sustained within the community. They are often intended to instigate relationships with the spirit world and with the magic and mystery of beliefs that bind the community and secure the future of the society. Examples include the first experience of certain sacred ceremonies, such as the first vision quest or the introduction into an *inipi* ceremony, the traditional Lakota sweat lodge.

Many traditions in our culture provide rites in socially accepted forms such as Bar and Bat Mitzvahs in the Jewish faith, or "coming out" parties for debutantes. Although these rites mark a major movement in one's life, they do not constitute initiation. Wilderness experiences for Boy Scouts and entrances into fraternal orders, however, are rites that can also be initiations, as are near-death experiences and the passage through a mental breakdown when one returns with a deeper comprehension of life's journey.

In some practices, such as Reiki, initiation is also used to confer specific awakenings or levels or formal degrees. In Alchemical Healing, *initiation* speaks of an event within which a shift or change occurs that accesses a new level of knowledge and experience, provides entry into an as yet unexplored dimension of awareness, or opens the way to previously inconceivable spiritual technology. The Journey to Thoth, during which one passes through the doorway of higher consciousness into the realm of Thoth for the first time, may constitute an initiation, especially if the relationships instituted are developed and become an integral part of one's life. Initiations can be ordeals but are not necessarily so.

In 1982 I had just taken my first Huna class with Nadia, whose initiations and teaching methods were entirely new to me. I could barely contain all the information, let alone comprehend the initiatory processes I had undergone. But the truth was that through the initiations, she had facilitated the rewiring of my energy channels to support a higher voltage and amperage of life force energy. She also took the class on several shamanic journeys in the form of guided visualizations. Although my experience during the journeys was not particularly noteworthy, the difference in my abilities as a healer became immediately evident.

I was in a deep sleep on the morning following that first class when I heard someone cry out my name. I crawled out of bed and went to the balcony to see who was calling me so early. Below stood a very distraught person, his face so distorted from swelling that it took me a moment to realize it was Tim, one of the carpenters who was working on a barn I was building at the time. He was suffering from an abscessed tooth that had kept him in agony throughout the night. He was scared and in pain, and could I help him? I pulled on some clothes and went down to take a closer look. It was not pretty. He could have given the elephant man a run for his money. One eye was swollen completely shut and his nose blended without a crease into his cheek. If I had been better educated about the gravity of his condition, I would have insisted he go to the emergency room immediately. I certainly suggested it, but he refused. He had a ferocious fear of dentists and had consumed about a quart of vodka during the night while attempting to fend off the fear and pain. Could I please help him?

My daughter Sage had joined us, and I was glad to have someone there for moral support. Tim sat on a bench in the garden and I began to work on him in the new way I had just learned, holding my hands over, but not touching, the skin. This was not because I had much confidence in my ability to use the new method—I didn't—but because I was afraid to touch him and it seemed like the only thing to do. It was very scary for me.

I centered myself, set a clear intention for healing, placed my hands over the distorted area on his face, and silently made a call for help. A strong current of energy began to flow through my hands; the electric, tingly feeling assured me that I was connected to the Universal Life Force.

Directing the light like laser beams off my fingertips, I simulated a small incision just above the abscessed tooth, then drew the surrounding field apart with my hands. Immediately I felt an opening and a deeper connection to the interior of his face, so I extended a more diffuse current of the energy off my fingertips with the intention of letting the traumatized area know I was there as a friend. It was as though I had long fingernails of light that went deep into the root source of his abscess, directly into the place of swelling and pain. I used these extensions of light to scoop up the poisons that were trapped in the abscess. Much to all our amazement, as I made the first pass and was lifting out what I can only describe as etheric gunk, Tim made a horrible grimace, turned his head to the side, and spat out a mouthful of yellow-green pus. It only took three or four passes to remove all the poison. We watched in astonishment as the swelling subsided and the pain vanished. When he went to the dentist on the following Monday, the tooth was removed without him having to take a course of antibiotics to alleviate infection.

Whether or not this healing experience can be attributed to the work I was doing at the same time is less important than that it happened at all. Maybe the abscess was ready to burst and it was a coincidence. The result was as important for me as it was for Tim, because I saw the potential of the new healing techniques I had just learned from Nadia. It also validated the power of initiation.

INITIATORY PROCESS OF THIS BOOK

The initiations you receive during the course of reading this book, if you choose to take them, are designed to create openings and to generate a new level of experience from which you can continue your work from a more expanded place than wherever you were when you started reading. They may introduce you into new dimensions of consciousness where power, intelligence, and additional frequencies of energy are available. Every person moves at his or her own pace, and the energies that are awakened will not exceed what an individual can handle. Your body has an energy system that is comparable to electrical wiring. You can carry more "juice" in accordance with the insulation that surrounds the wires. Attunements and initiatory journeys help prepare your system to handle a greater volume of energy, or a specific frequency. If you have already had similar adjustments from another system, you will be able to recognize the additional power and subtle alterations that these initiations provide.

No one system is necessarily better than another, and there is no reason that the system of Alchemical Healing should not be compatible with whatever other methods of healing you are using. Although I believe that metaphysical laws are consistent, different traditions have different ways of expressing how these laws operate. For example, the perception of chakra systems varies in different disciplines: chakras might be named or placed differently in the body depending on who is describing them. Each system has its own integrity and is correct from its point of view. In Alchemical Healing we work with five elements, including Earth, Water, Fire, Air, and Akasha (spirit or ether). Chinese acupuncture uses five elements also, but their system includes Water, Fire, Air, Wood, and Metal. One is not better than the other, they are simply different, and used in a different context.

All of the initiations can be repeated from time to time to

strengthen your connections; however, once the connections are made, they last for a lifetime. When you have accessed the Universal Life Force from its infinite source, it will always be available to you, as will the elements, spirit guides, and totems. Each repeat simply reinforces the original experience—and often contributes something new and unexpected.

THOTH

The first initiation we will undertake is the introduction and connection to Thoth. Thoth is the guide and teacher for Alchemical Healing, our muse. Also known as Djehuti, he is one of the most important gods in the Egyptian pantheon. He is a moon god, and is concerned with the measuring and ordering of life as well as wisdom, language, communication, healing, sciences, writing, magic, and more. He is also prominent in his role as scribe. He keeps the records of our soul's journey. To the ancient Egyptians, he represented the highest concept of mind, most closely resembling the Greek concept of Logos.

It is important to note that Thoth expresses a quality of consciousness and awareness that we are all attempting to attain. When we are in touch with Thoth, we are in touch with the wisest level of our own mind, the most discerning perspective accessible to us. It is important to address, here at the outset, that when we are speaking of deities, archetypes, or animal totems—any of the allies we work with—we are connecting with aspects of our own nature, qualities that are part of the collective consciousness of which we are a part.

The sacred ibis is Thoth's most prevailing totemic image, although he also appears as the dog-faced baboon and, in certain functions, as a cobra. He is usually seen with a man's body and the head of an ibis wearing the lunar disk. (As his solar self he appears as a baboon with the sun disk on his head.) The ibis is a fisher bird that lives in the marshes along the Nile where papyrus grows. Fish are an ancient symbol of knowledge, and papyrus was used to make the scrolls upon which the scribes of ancient Egypt kept many of their records. The ibis, being a most intelligent bird, is associated with the element Air and thus with the mind, communication, and humor.

Although we think of Thoth as Egyptian, there are many myths and stories that speak of him from as far back as legendary Atlantis, and his attributes were often associated with Hermes in Greece and with Mercury in Roman times. Throughout history, Thoth has been honored as the impeccable teacher's teacher, the one who brought wisdom and civilization to people. He is the mediator of the *neteru,* the cosmic principles who make up the Egyptian pantheon.

Thoth was always called upon when things got too far out of balance. It was he who replaced the head of Isis with that of a cow, when the enraged Horus cut it off during a battle with his uncle Set. And when Set gouged out Horus's eye, it was Thoth who gave Horus a new one, the all-seeing Eye of Horus. Thoth also bestowed words of power upon the goddess Isis, and taught her the magic for which she is renowned.

Many modern and ancient spiritual traditions have their source in Thoth, including the Western magical traditions and, according to some, the Masons, the Cabala, and the Tarot. Difficulties occur if the teachings are held rigid, bound by rules and reiterated with exactitude, because they become stilted and their integrity is corrupted. Or they are watered down through assimilation into the main stream of consciousness, losing their sacredness and their edge.

Alchemical Healing, as a body of work, is greater in sum than in the parts that brought it into form. It finds its source in an ancient lineage of Thoth. This lineage maintains its power without the levels of secrecy and rigid structure that limit access to many esoteric traditions. A person does not have to be part of the lineage to be a practitioner of Alchemical Healing. When presented in a teaching context, however, the initiations and activations should be performed by those in the lineage because they have been given the technical and spiritual connections that make them work. Every person has the inborn capacity to connect to source directly. Teachers of Alchemical Healing, by virtue of their soul's experience and the skills gained in life while fulfilling their service, bear witness to and facilitate this process. They hold specific maps of consciousness and relationships with spiritual entities with whom they co-create and facilitate as a team. If in the course of working with this book you feel called to teach Alchemical Healing, connect directly with me or with one of the teachers listed in Appendix II.

The more we practice Alchemical Healing, the more we see our intentions manifest in the patterns of our lives. When a person has fully integrated this body of work into his life and being, it goes through a metamorphosis, and the resulting permutation is expressed through the adept's own form of healing or transformational work. This keeps the teachings alive and vibrant through constant renewal, although the founding principles remain intact.

Medieval alchemy was considered the Royal Art. Alchemical Healing is also an art form, and so its practitioners have the freedom to express themselves in the style that develops as uniquely theirs. The palette for Alchemical Healing includes many aspects of energy and light, as well as the basic elements of the creation in both the material and spirit worlds. Everything has intelligence and spirit, and all can be brought to assist with their unique perspective and gifts.

You will journey to Thoth through an alchemical process that safely takes you into the perception of higher consciousness. I recommend that you have someone read the journey to you, or make a tape in your own voice and play it back. Ellipses (. . .) in the text indicate that time is required to develop your inner perception. It works best if you have a pause button handy so that when you come to the pauses you can extend them for as long as you need. A third option is to simply read the journey slowly—closing your eyes between each instruction—and visualize, listen, and feel the result before continuing.

The purpose of the following journey is to meet—and begin to develop a relationship with—your High Self, the wisest aspect of your being, as expressed through Thoth. Thoth will continue to appear as a principle guide as you progress in learning Alchemical Healing. He will be available to answer questions and inform your experience throughout.

Those readers who have been previously initiated to Thoth through my work may choose to begin with the journey in the next chapter, the Journey of Commitment.

As solemn as this occasion may seem, be prepared to be surprised. Thoth often shares his gifts with great humor, imbuing each challenging level of development with a mirthful measure of joy. Just now as I was taking my husband on the journey to make sure I have it written correctly, Thoth showed up as Groucho Marx, an obvious admonishment not to take ourselves too seriously.

It is my greatest privilege to introduce Thoth to my readers, because when you develop a relationship with this great teacher, he will present you with experiences that not only allow you to learn, but also allow you to become wise about whatever you are learning.

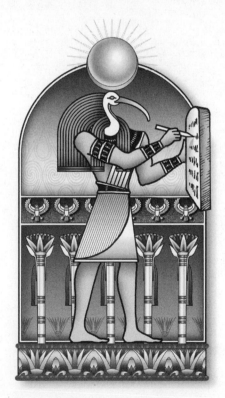

Figure 5.1. Thoth

INITIATION

JOURNEY TO THOTH

Relax, close your eyes, and breathe deeply. Fill your body with the nourishing breath of life. With each breath you become more grounded and more centered. . . .

Place your hands before you with the palms facing upward.

You will receive the gift of a purple-black egg, flecked in gold. This is an etheric egg, a spirit egg, an egg of creation . . .

Draw the egg into your abdomen. Feel as it nestles comfortably inside you . . .

Bring your attention to your heart center. Within your heart dwells the eternal flame of your being. As you bring your heart flame into focus, direct love and your flame will grow. See, feel, imagine, or know as your flame intensifies . . . as it brightens and grows . . . as it sends warmth and light throughout your entire being. . . .

A crown is placed on your head. Notice what your crown is made of and how it feels. . . . This crown marks this empowerment and provides the doorway through which your consciousness travels as you journey using this alchemical pathway.

Bring your attention now to where the egg has been gestating in your abdomen. As you focus on the egg, its outer shell is absorbed into your abdominal wall, revealing a cauldron, a golden vessel, filled with the primordial waters of life. As you observe this vessel, it expands to fill the space of your abdomen. . . .

The spirit of a healing herb is placed within your cauldron. Allow a moment for it to steep, releasing its essence into the waters within. . . .

Begin to stir the waters of life in your golden cauldron. As you stir these waters, they begin to rise. . . . Continue to stir up the waters, and as they are uplifted, they will meet the fire in your heart. . . . You might even hear the hissing, bubbling, crackling

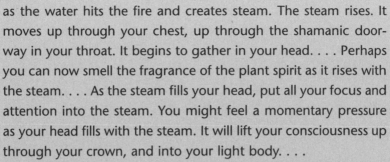

as the water hits the fire and creates steam. The steam rises. It moves up through your chest, up through the shamanic doorway in your throat. It begins to gather in your head. . . . Perhaps you can now smell the fragrance of the plant spirit as it rises with the steam. . . . As the steam fills your head, put all your focus and attention into the steam. You might feel a momentary pressure as your head fills with the steam. It will lift your consciousness up through your crown, and into your light body. . . .

Look to your left and you will see Thoth, in whatever form he presents himself. If you do not see him, feel, imagine, or simply know his presence. He will come around to stand before you. . . .

Greet Thoth with respect. If you are visual and see him, make eye contact and open your heart. . . .

He is glad to see you. He has much to share. You can ask questions, or simply stay open to receive any messages that he has for you at this time. The messages may not be verbal. Notice any activity. . . . Look for the hidden meanings. The longer you stay the more details you will receive. . . .

When you feel that this experience is complete for this time, be sure to thank Thoth. . . .

He will assist you back into your physical body and ordinary consciousness through the doorway that is your crown. . . .

Be sure to ground and center yourself before opening your eyes. . .

In order to return to Thoth for further guidance, you can do an abbreviated form of this alchemical process, because once you have been given the cauldron it is not necessary to do that part again. You will find that with enough practice, you'll be able to make this alteration in your perception with ease, ultimately finding Thoth effortlessly in the light of your radiant heart flame.

You can visit Thoth whenever you have questions, the more specific the better.

6
COMMITMENT

ONE OF THE STRONGEST motivators for the Alchemical Healing work is commitment. It is one thing to acknowledge that there is suffering and pain in this world, and it is quite another to do something about it. Those of us who have responded to the call to heal are honoring a deep commitment, more or less consciously. Those who recognize suffering and want to choose to be part of the solutions rather than part of the problems can start by making a commitment to serve the healing of the planet and all of its creatures. That commitment itself will serve to attract the tools you require in order to fulfill your intention.

The more you ritualize your commitment, the stronger the force in your life will be that will direct you to the appropriate tools. As I review my own life and prayers, I can remember some of the sequence that started with the first time I prayed with the sacred Pipe for clarity, for the ability to surrender and to become a servant for the healing of the planet and its inhabitants. As my journey progressed I began to see myself committed as a seeker of truth, then as a healer, and more recently as a teacher with a voice advocating for wisdom and personal empowerment. Although my commitment has changed from time to time, it has stayed fundamentally the same since I first realized that we, the people of the earth, had made a mess of things and no one is going to show up to clean it up for us. We have to do it ourselves. I have seen associates focus their specific intentions on creating healing for the children or for abused women, writing a book, or healing the environment. Their success in developing their life's work is directly related to their level of commitment.

It is all too easy to fall prey to helplessness in view of the challenges that are facing us. There is always the temptation to see ourselves as victims, with no potential to make a difference. There is no power to that, and no joy. When we are functioning in resonance with our divine purpose, each moment is new, rich, and filled with vitality. And it starts with our commitment.

A good method to state your commitment is in the presence of a witness. In the practice of Alchemical Healing, that witness takes the form of Thoth. When you ritualize your commitment in the presence of Thoth he records your statement in the record of your soul, marking the moment in the indelible stone of your story—a contract that is probably more remembered than newly created.

This commitment is not about becoming a great Alchemical Healer; it is about becoming receptive to any aspect of your potential that you may have missed, or that you are ready to embrace. It is about your reason for being in this life, on this planet, at this time.

For the purposes of this work, I recommend creating a ritual within which you can make your commitment. To accomplish this, you must first determine precisely *what* you are committing to. What do you want to be when you grow up? Given that you are reading this book, you may wish to become a healer, or work toward better health in your own life. Perhaps you've been working in a corporation, yet dream of becoming a writer or an artist. You might discover latent talents later in life, and find that you would benefit by returning to school. Be willing to accept that you may have to give up certain things in order to move forward toward your goals. Committing to personal growth, development, and transformation can also be worthy objectives. I suggest you be as specific as possible, and make your choice something you are willing to honor through thick and thin while you are achieving your committed goal.

Take the time you need to clarify your intention, and write down what you come up with. Journaling the process will yield a good source for future reflection.

CREATING A RITUAL

To expend the time and energy to create ritual is in itself a statement of commitment. Attention is a form of currency, one of great value in any spiritual activity. The strength and power of ritual is in direct relationship to the focus and concentration of the participants.

Creating an altar can enhance rituals, although it is not absolutely necessary. The spirit world is nourished by your attention, and an altar provides a focal point for the spirit(s) that you are welcoming. To create an altar, set aside a small space on a mantel, table, or even a windowsill. Place on it a candle and an object that symbolizes your commitment, such as a stone or crystal that will remind you of this event. The altar does not have to be elaborate, though fetishes, statuary, or images of allies, deities, or spirit guides that you would like to invoke can add a welcoming environment.

It is also important to smudge with the smoke of cedar, sage, sweet grass, or incense as a means of purification and to clear your mind before starting your ritual. If scent is unavailable or offensive in some way, you can call on the spirit of sage to purify the area.

An essential aspect of any ritual is the invocation of your spirit guides, ancestors, and whoever else you want present from the spirit world to witness the event. I always call and honor the powers of the four cardinal directions, plus the powers of Above and Earth. At the end of the calling, I like to offer cornmeal because it is a symbol of the nourishing fruits of life. If it is not possible to do the invocation out of doors where you can sprinkle the cornmeal on the earth, you can use a receptacle for your offering.

INVOKING THE DIRECTIONS

One of the simplest ways to center yourself is to note where you are in relation to the cardinal directions. It is an instant way to place yourself in the center of the universe and to orient yourself accordingly.

Every place I travel, every different tribe or culture I encounter has its own way of perceiving the powers of the directions. None is more right than the others and all can be incorporated as appropriate in the moment. It is important that you feel the rightness of whatever or whomever you associate with a direction, and that can only come with practice.

Some people prefer to make their call out loud to include the power of their voice; some offer it silently, inwardly; others choose to sing it. My own invocations change from time to time, according to the intention and style of the work of the moment. I might call different entities while doing work in Egypt than when I am at home or in Peru. Different cultures start with different directions, though most seem to start in the East; some go clockwise, some counter-clockwise, and some in a cross. I might start a Pipe ceremony in the West because of the way I was initially taught. The East is the most common direction for starting because the sun rises in the East. Yet there are times when I am drawn to start with the ancestors in the North. It is most important to feel for yourself what is appropriate unless you are adhering to a specific tradition.

My call to the directions is associated with the elements: Air to the East, Fire to the South, Water to the West, and Earth to the North. Usually I call six directions, including Above and Below, and sometimes I add a seventh for Within or Great Spirit, or Great Spirit that dwells within. If I am asked to participate in a ceremony based on a specific tradition, I adhere as best I can to the tenets of that tradition. The archetypes also change spontaneously from time to time, depending upon the work of the moment. Feel free to use the following invocation until your own generates from your inner being.

INVOCATION

Hail to the powers of the East. Hail to the sun that rises each day to give light and energy into my life. I call the winged ones, the eagle and the hawk, the condor and the vulture. I invite you to come into this ceremony. May the powers of the East give me clear sight and illuminate my way that I might see clearly my path on my journey here on Mother Earth. I honor you. I welcome you. I give thanks for your presence.

Hail to the powers of the South, where the sun is at its zenith. I call the lioness and the puma, the jaguar and the leopard—I call on all who represent the fire of life. Come into this ceremony, give passion to my every thought and deed. Doctoring and helping spirits of the South, come into this circle that all present may receive the help they need to heal themselves and one another. I honor and welcome you. I thank you for your presence.

Hail to the powers of the West, the place of introspection and of the hidden mysteries. I call Anubis, guardian of the underworld. Protect us in our work, show us the pathways that move from the darkness into the light. I call the bear, bringer of dreams, and all who dwell in the waters of the world. I honor Kuan Yin and Mary, and all the goddesses of compassion—come into our circle that we might know kindness and mercy. I honor you and welcome you. I thank you for your presence.

Hail to the powers of the North, the direction of the keepers of wisdom. I call the ancestors, with gratitude for the symbols and signs you have left along the way for us. I call White Buffalo Woman with gratitude for her wisdom, her strength, and the nourishment of life. I honor and welcome all the powers of the North, and I give thanks for your presence.

Hail to the beings Above, sky beings, celestial ones, thunder beings, Thoth and Maät, spirit guides and intelligent beings throughout the universe; I call you. I honor you. I pray for a clearer connection with the guidance that comes from Above, so that I may walk in balance in my journey here on Mother Earth. I welcome you and thank you for your presence in my life and at this ceremony.

Hail to Mother Earth. Thank you for my body and my life. Thank you for all my relatives with whom I share this wondrous planet. I call on your powers, the powers of the elements, the stones and the plants, and all who walk, swim, crawl, and fly. Please send your powers into this ceremony, for it is dedicated to the healing of Mother Earth and All Our Relations.

Hail to the Center of my being, where I am united with all life, Great Spirit without and within. May I always remember the beauty and love that dwells in my heart.

As I am directing my call, facing each direction, I offer a small pinch of cornmeal in my extended hand. At the end of the invocation I pour the cornmeal on the ground or into a receptacle that I can later take outside and offer to nature. I offer my prayer and/or intention to the Great Mystery or Creator of all. Use whatever name most suits your image of the divine. Then continue into the ritual or ceremony.

The following journey begins with the abbreviated alchemy, which can be used to open your connection to Thoth at the beginning of any of the initiations and exercises presented in the rest of the book. You can also use this abbreviated alchemy at any other time that you wish to connect with Thoth.

INITIATION

JOURNEY OF COMMITMENT

Relax, close your eyes, and breathe deeply. Fill your body with the nourishing breath of life. With each breath you become more grounded and more centered. . . .

Devote attention to your heart flame, directing love to make it grow and spread its radiance throughout your being, filling you with warmth and light. . . .

Stir the waters within your golden cauldron. . . . Notice as the waters rise to meet the flame in your heart. . . . Listen for the hissing, bubbling, and crackling sounds as the water meets the fire and turns to steam. . . .

The steam rises, opening the shamanic passageway at your throat and filling your head. Place your entire attention within the steam. As it gathers in your head, it will lift your consciousness up through your crown and into your light body. . . .

Thoth comes around from your left. . . .

[Proceed with the Journey of Commitment.]

Greet Thoth with respect. Take a moment to see, hear, feel, or know his presence. Make eye contact and open your heart, asking for help and guidance as you learn this healing form as a means of helping yourself, others, and the planet. . . .

Awaken all your senses to perceive Thoth and receive his response—see, feel, know, and hear his presence. Allow time to receive whatever message or information he has for you. . . .

Upon assent, in whatever way it comes, offer your commitment. Speak it aloud with the power of your will and intention. Thoth will acknowledge and record your commitment. . . .

Thoth has something further to share with you. You will be given an experience and a tool or special adjustment that is personal and just for you. You may also receive some instructions as to how to proceed on your spiritual path. . . .

Take a moment to further develop the relationship you are forming with Thoth. It is okay to ask a question if one comes to you at this time. . . .

Be sure to thank Thoth. . . .

Thoth will assist you back into your physical body and ordinary consciousness through the doorway that is your crown. . . .

Be sure to ground and center yourself, and thank and release those entities and the directions that you have called in to witness. . . .

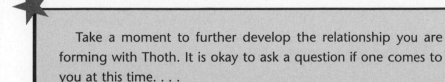

It is advisable to take a few moments at the end of each journey or practice to be still and quiet, in order to integrate your experience and to record it in your journal.

7
FORGIVENESS

FORGIVENESS IS A FUNDAMENTAL PROCESS on the path of Alchemical Healing, as it is in Huna and other spiritual traditions. When I began to study Huna in 1982, the first subject we dealt with was forgiveness, for good reason: it cleared the way for a larger current of energy to flow through us.

It takes effort to hold on to old guilt, grief, and pain, just as grudges and gripes contribute to stress. *For-giving* is what takes us back to before the giving of the hurt. Or consider it as that which is required before we can give fully of ourselves. Forgiveness is releasing rather than accepting. It frees up energy that has been holding stressful patterns in place. When we truly forgive, we release those tightly held patterns and can access more energy.

There are many ways to approach forgiveness and many rituals to achieve it. Ritual reinforces the subconscious mind's sense of what is real. When we ritualize the act of forgiveness, the effect is reflected in our real-time relationships, regardless of whether the other person is aware on a conscious level of the work we have done.

A very important key to healing work is to understand that we are directly connected to whatever we are thinking about. Whether we think about an inanimate object, a distant friend or acquaintance, an ancestor, or someone with whom we are in close and loving relationship, our thoughts connect us like a complex weaving. If I'm speaking of it, thinking of it, or looking at it, I'm connected to it. We weave the tapestry of our lives just as spiders create their webs. In our thoughts, we are constantly spinning our connections to everything around us.

There's a Hawaiian word, *aka,* which, though possibly not related to the Sanskrit word *akasha,* bears a resemblance to it in sound and meaning. It refers to the essence of the material on which our thoughts ride, the threads with which we spin our interconnections. The tiny filaments of aka that we spin with each thought become more and more numerous as our relationships develop, and the threads are spun into cords. The multidimensional fabric of our lives is woven and given texture by these fine filaments, threads, and cords that we constantly emanate and receive as we interact with our surroundings.

In our loving relationships the cords are luminous and vibrant, and energy moves freely between, helping us to be mutually supportive. When there is anguish, pain, or misery in a relationship, what started out as luminous fibers turn dark and dense, which prevents the free-flowing exchange of energy. The thickness, texture, and weight of these cords, as well as the movement of light and energy through them, are directly related to the quality of the relationship, or in some cases, the trauma associated with the relationship. Instead of being mutually supportive, a relationship can become weighted down like a tree with many dead branches. We carry that weight with us and use up a great deal of our energy just to support it. It is actually no different than natural law in the plant world. Prune your apple tree, removing the dead wood to make space for new growth, and your tree will respond with renewed vigor.

We can imagine ourselves as a tree. The spinal column is like the tree trunk, and the main branches extend from the chakra centers. Each chakra center is associated with an element and specific issues related to the elemental significance of that chakra. The cording occurs in accordance with the issues around each level. In complex relationships, such as those between parents and children and other people who are close, the cords exist in several centers, possibly even in all of them. Cords representing other specific relationships can be found at the relevant chakra centers. For example, a cord might connect you with a teacher at the fifth center because the throat chakra relates to communication. Your supervisor at work might turn up at the root chakra where security and survival issues are located, or at the third chakra, where personal power issues appear.

Each person's tree of life is the source of the personal tapestry woven by these threads of different qualities and thicknesses, textures, weights, and colors. Sometimes the tree needs pruning. What pruning shears can we use to rid ourselves of the old, dense, brittle cords, the limbs that don't serve us anymore? The answer is forgiveness.

Forgiveness is an amazing thing. With it, you can transform darkness into luminosity. Or you can simply release a cord altogether. You don't have to worry about losing your connections to people; even if you release a cord, you can always build a new one, and hope that the new ones will sustain their luminosity. This alchemical process is fundamental to our work as healers. It is much the same as turning lead into gold.

Forgiveness goes in two directions. Sometimes it is appropriate for you to forgive others, and at other times you need to ask for the forgiveness of the person at the other end of the cord. Or you can ask the person what it would take for him or her to forgive you. Be willing to negotiate for that forgiveness. Sometimes you will find yourself at both ends of the cord, and you must give yourself the same forgiveness that you give others.

The chakra centers are energetic portals, points of power through which you, as an individual, access realms of consciousness related to the elements and basic issues of life. They are arranged much like a ladder of consciousness, starting with the tailbone. Most of the chakras are in alignment with the spinal column as it rises upward through the body.

As you proceed through your life you are constantly weaving a multidimensional lattice of aka. The threads originate at each of your chakra centers according to the element and issues associated with that chakra. By understanding this model, you can perceive how various issues—physical, emotional, spiritual, and mental (along with their corresponding elements)—are linked to your physical body and can be recognized, nurtured, and healed accordingly.

The accompanying illustration (Figure 7.1) and expanded descriptions provide a way of perceiving the relationships between the chakras and issues that contribute to both your illness and your well-being. They suggest where to look for cords associated with specific situations and people when you perform the forgiveness ritual that follows. Because so much of our culture has become drug dependent, I am including some of the substances rampant in our society that affect the chakras. Substance abuse almost always results in cording that requires forgiveness. Even a single substance-related event can block the free flow of energy. For example, an embarrassing moment that occurred when you were drunk may be siphoning energy if it is still unresolved.

1. The root chakra is located at the base of the spine. It is associated with the element Earth, and is related to all things physical, including physical healing. The issues you will encounter here are often associated with survival, security, fight or flight responses, trust, and material support. Family members such as parents may be strongly present at the first chakra center, not only because they brought you into this life, but because they were integral to your security as a young and dependent person. Manifestation, including abundance and lack, are also associated with the first chakra. The substances that most affect the root chakra in our society are opiates, depressants, and hypnotics. When used in excess, those drugs compromise our basic fight-or-flight responses and our survival instincts.

2. The second chakra is located in the area of the genitals/womb. It is associated with the element Water. Emotional issues are found here, as are issues concerning reproduction, nurturing, sexuality and sexual relationships, children, sensitivity, and the social pecking order. Cording regarding relationships, jealousy,

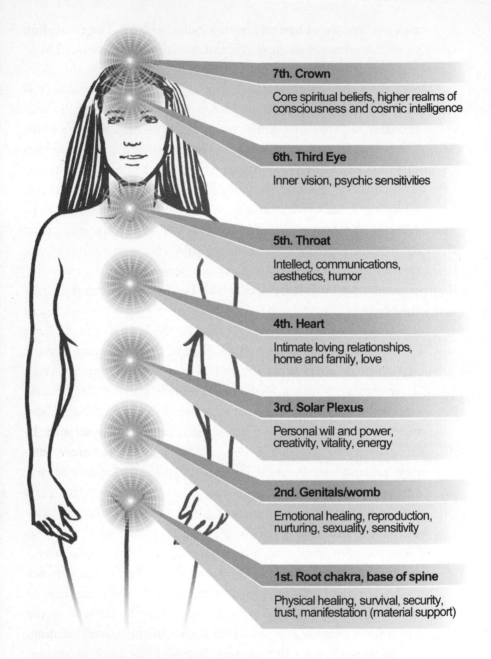

7th. Crown

Core spiritual beliefs, higher realms of consciousness and cosmic intelligence

6th. Third Eye

Inner vision, psychic sensitivities

5th. Throat

Intellect, communications, aesthetics, humor

4th. Heart

Intimate loving relationships, home and family, love

3rd. Solar Plexus

Personal will and power, creativity, vitality, energy

2nd. Genitals/womb

Emotional healing, reproduction, nurturing, sexuality, sensitivity

1st. Root chakra, base of spine

Physical healing, survival, security, trust, manifestation (material support)

Figure 7.1. The Chakras and the Issues Related to Each

and our territorial nature are also included here. The prevailing substance in our society that influences this center is alcohol.

3. The third chakra is located at the solar plexus. This chakra is associated with the element Fire, and is concerned with one's personal will and power. It includes issues around one's identity, motivation, vitality, and action. Some of the darker issues connected to this chakra involve power over others, destructive behavior, rage, and violence. Nicotine, cocaine, amphetamines, and caffeine are ubiquitous in our society. They are often abused and, consequently, may affect a person's will, thus affecting the third chakra center.

4. The heart is the center of our being. The heart chakra stands between the three lower chakras (each of which is grounded in the terrestrial laws of physics) and the three upper chakras (through which we connect to the universal or collective mind). The heart is the platform from which we move from a dualistic approach to life to a view of the multiplicity of possibilities. The intelligence of the heart, recognized in ancient Egypt and many mystical cultures, is now being validated by science. In the heart center we find issues related to love, our most intimate relationships, mating for life and progeny, and the domestic issues around home and family. Our clearest guidance is heart centered. Chocolate and MDMA are drugs that are associated with the heart.

5. The fifth, or throat, chakra is associated with the element Air. Communications, sound, art, humor, and aesthetics are all accessed through this center. Teachers may be present at the fifth center because it is related to communication and learning. The fifth chakra is the shamanic doorway, the narrow passage through which each person must travel alone. It connects our dual, either/or reality with the larger collective reality in which there are infinite possibilities. In our culture the most widely

used substance that affects this center is marijuana. Yoga, martial arts, music, and initiatory practices affect all the centers but have a particularly strong effect on the fifth and above.

6. The third eye, or sixth chakra center, is where all of the elements come together to support each person's inner vision of reality. Because all of our senses meet here, it is a primary point of power that we can develop through yogic disciplines or martial arts, and other advanced practices found in various traditions. This center is also affected by psychedelic substances, including sacred plant medicines such as peyote, mushrooms, San Pedro, ibogane, ayahuasca, and so forth. It should be noted that we can affect all of the centers through conscious intention and focus, breathing, and both physical and spiritual exercise. Here cords relate to our psychic perceptions in the spirit realms, and perhaps to psychic interference.

7. The seventh center, the crown chakra, is located at the top of the head and can be reached through the fontanel, a point on the brow between the third eye and the crown. It is associated with the element Akasha and when it is opened we can have direct access to the superconscious mind, also known as the upper world or High Self. Issues at this chakra are generally associated with spiritual or religious belief systems and with access to higher realms of consciousness, including extraterrestrial and other cosmic intelligence. Both the lower or inner world of the collective unconsciousness and the higher world of the superconscious mind are accessible through inner travel—you have to go in to get out. There are usually very few cords here, and the only dark ones are likely to be associated with betrayals of faith or shattering of fundamental beliefs.

★ ☽ ★

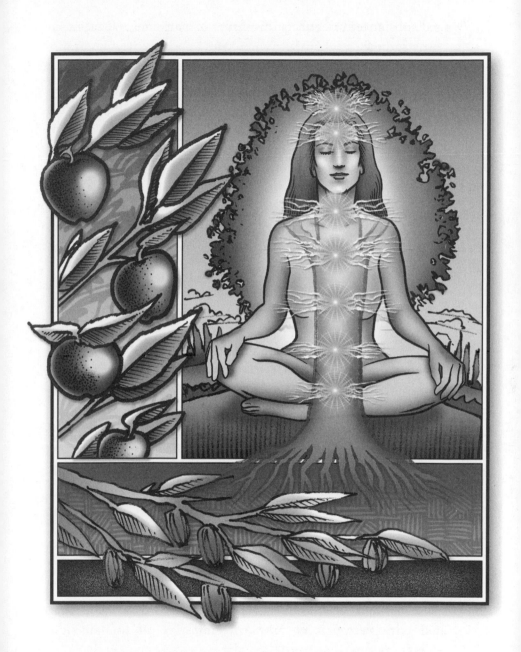

Figure 7.2. Forgiveness Meditation

What follows is an exercise that can help you to prune and maintain your own sacred tree of life. When you have removed or transformed the dead weight of dense and dark cords, you will have more energy to apply more constructively in your life. Once you have cleared yourself of all the unwanted attachments, it is easy to maintain this state by being conscious and forgiving in the moment, rather than allowing dark and heavy cords to gain hold whenever any of the issues arise again.

When you do the exercise, you will be able to perceive the cords that exist between you and others. You will be able to follow those cords to their source, at which point you will encounter the people and situations with whom you have issues that you need to resolve through forgiveness. Then you will have the opportunity to prune your sacred tree by directly offering forgiveness to or requesting forgiveness from the High Self of the person with whom you are connected.

It is important to remember that some of the cords are likely to lead back to you. We are often hardest on ourselves, and we require the same forgiveness for ourselves as for others. Allow some time for contemplation before beginning this exercise, and be prepared to do it again and again until you find yourself clear of blockages in your energy system based on this model. Once you have cleared your dense cords and have only luminous connections, you'll need to revisit this process from time to time to maintain a free-flowing exchange between you and those with whom you continue to relate.

EXERCISE
Forgiveness Meditation

Close your eyes and ground and center.

See yourself as a transparent being. Focus your attention along the vertical alignment at the central core of your being, which may appear as the trunk of your sacred tree. Seek the sensations that identify the chakra centers. You may perceive them as luminous wheels of light. Take the time you need to allow these images to become strong and clear, in whatever way they develop. That may be through feelings, thoughts, knowing, or images, or your own personal and unique perception. . . .

Begin by focusing on the first wheel of light at the first chakra center at the base of your spine. Look there for the threads and cords that emanate like branches or twigs. You will see lots of connections, many of which are luminous and some of which are dark and dense or brittle. Reach in with your inner hand to remove those dark cords that come away easily.

Choose one of the dense cords that remain, and follow it to its source. There you will get a picture or thought of the person at the other end of the cord. When you perceive the being at the other end, you will know whether you must offer forgiveness or ask for it.

Open your heart as best you can. . . . Offer forgiveness by saying in your mind to the person, "I forgive you completely." . . .

If you feel you need forgiveness from the person at the other end of the cord, ask what you can do to be forgiven, and be willing to negotiate. . . .

Notice as the dark and dense cord that connects you either vanishes or turns clear and luminous. . . .

Work your way up through the chakra system from the first to the seventh chakra, dealing with as many cords as is reasonable and comfortable.

When you have dealt with as many of the cords as you are able to at the moment, release the image you have created and ground and center yourself. Notice how much lighter you feel.

You can return to complete the work over a period of time, after which maintaining clear chakras is easily accomplished by checking in and doing the exercise periodically.

8
HEALING ENERGY BASICS

IN ORDER TO PRACTICE Alchemical Healing, you need to develop awareness and sensitivity to energy, the ubiquitous force that animates the material world. Movement is energy. Emotion is energy. To some who cannot see it or feel it, it may not appear to exist. Yet even the most insensitive person can see energy rising from pavement on a blistering day. And we all know when we are lacking in energy, for without it we cannot function.

Energy is defined by the physical and functional characteristics of how it behaves. Energy is active—it is constantly in motion. It heats our houses and runs our cars. Energy not only changes inert matter, either by moving it, stopping it, or changing its direction, it also animates our emotions and our passion.

As one works with Alchemical Healing, one's relationship to and understanding of energy is likely to change. The life force that permeates everything and everybody becomes a working ally rather than an observed phenomenon.

Physicists recognize that the universe contains infinite potential energy. In order to manifest that potential for healing, we need only use the tools of awareness and visualization described in this book. Energy is easily moved with intention, and flows through the interconnected, ever-changing patterns that make up the whole of creation. When our minds envision color, shape, or movement, the energy responds.

The power of our healing work comes from this understanding of energy: we can effect form intentionally by developing our thoughts with imagination, will, and focused attention, and by engaging our senses. The subtle, intangible energies we use in healing are malleable, and if our awareness is trained to sense them, we can mold those energies into tangible, substantial form.

When we work with the energy fields that surround life forms, such as the auric field around a person, we affect a more basic reality than the physical, and as a result, the physical is invited to change. Matter is an end product of the process of giving form to energy. Although we work at an earlier stage of the process of manifestation, when you change the level of the energy, there is a physical effect that you can witness. Consider the process of ice turning to water, and then to steam.

Just as intelligence permeates the universe, energy itself is infused with consciousness, vitalizing the tapestry of life and informing the patterns that connect all things. We are all connected, and we are all affected by the acts and thoughts of others. Life forms that grow in colonies, such as coral, fungi, and ants, exemplify the cooperative effort that produces many individuals as part of a whole. In actuality, all life is composed of cooperative and symbiotic relationships, because energy at its basis is love.

The energy that vitalizes matter is imbued with intelligence that is cooperating to create matter. Simply allowing energy to move through you and out your hands into another form will create an effect. That is its purpose and its joy. With the addition of intention, you give this energy direction (marching orders). We have the opportunity to exercise our choice to empower and direct energy for healing.

A good parallel example can be found in the practice of the

martial arts, tai chi and qigong. As the practitioner puts out the call, the energy comes in, focuses and intensifies, often raising the physical temperature of the body of the person, or of the specific place in the body where the energy is being directed. It is most important to develop and attune your abilities to visualize and to focus your awareness and intention through practice.

It must be noted that energy does not moralize. The power to change things is dangerous when wielded by one who is not in service to the needs of the people and the creation. When we set out to change things, even in healing, we must always take care to examine the possible consequences of our actions, and keep ourselves clear and centered. That said, we cannot be attached to the result of our healing work because we do not decide the form in which healing happens. That is decided by all the consciousness involved, including the one who is receiving the healing. Although the same is true when you intend harm—that harm is only received if there is an acceptance of and permission for it to manifest—you are still responsible for your own intentions.

As you develop skill in healing, you will come to realize that it is not possible to act unilaterally, because we are all connected—we are all one. Healing as a creative process is a cooperative venture, the work of a collaborative team that brings about more than the original intention of the instigating healer, and usually surpasses it. A healer who clings to an expectation will be disappointed and will not perceive that her motivating intention has spawned something beyond her original imagining. When you invoke a healing process with this work, you are the person who is presenting an idea to a collective—yourself, your spirit allies, and the higher self of the person you are working with. The collective fulfills that idea in its own way, and what manifests surpasses your idea and is in harmony with the intentions and consciousness of all involved.

As you focus your attention on energy, it begins to reveal itself in various forms. You can walk into a room of people and in an instant know a great deal about them because of an energetic connection that you feel. Certainly, when you are in the presence of deep love, sexual attraction, or acute repulsion, you have instinctive awareness of energy at work. It becomes palpable, tangible. At times it seems as though you could "cut it with a knife." When you have more energy, you get more work done. On the other hand, when energy is blocked, it stagnates and is hard to move. By involving yourself in practices such as yoga, martial arts, or healing, you honor and develop a more conscious relationship with the subtle energies that move through us all—and you keep them flowing.

Try rubbing your hands together quickly for a moment, and feel the heat that is created from the friction. Continue rubbing for another moment; then hold your hands about twelve inches apart facing each other. Slowly bring them together. What do you notice? Can you feel the pressure as the auric field that surrounds each hand presses upon the other? Does it tingle? Does it feel warm or energetic? Is there a thickness? A tangibility? The energy that you have stimulated is a palpable force that you can develop and direct, and, ultimately, use to effect healing.

There are many ways to raise or develop energy for healing. Rubbing the hands together can certainly give a person the feel of it. Just doing that simple exercise—and directing the energy in your palms toward wherever you wish to send it—can create change. In fact, this is a good way for the uninitiated to begin to experience energy and its movement. You can easily feel its transmission by putting your hands on your own body, especially if you direct it to a place that is in pain.

Our bodies function somewhat like batteries. We expend energy and then recharge through eating, resting, and exercising. When we are in emotional crisis or even near it, we feel drained. Healing energy, on the other hand, comes through you, not from you. Our physical bodies exist in layers of subtle energy fields, called *auras,* which extend out from our physical form. Those who "see" auras, either naturally or through training, can be informed by the color and animation evident within these subtle bodies. These fields provide information about the physical, emotional, mental, and even spiritual status of an individual. That information can be useful in diagnosis of disease. Often the information in one's auric field pre-cedes the actual physical manifestation of illness or healing.

The clearer your energy field is, the easier it is for the subtle ener-gies to pass through your body, and the better attuned you are to receive them. No matter how much training we have, if we allow static or corrosion to interfere with our connection to source, we will not have access to the fullness of our resources. In this way we are similar to an automobile battery: when the cable gets corroded, the charge cannot get through. If the conduit is kept clean, then we will be more successful at whatever we attempt.

Energy also exists within things, in accordance with their power. You can see energy surrounding plants and trees, even people, espe-cially if you sit with them and defocus your eyes. There is a very sub-tle glow, a radiance of life that surrounds all living things. When you focus on that surrounding field, you can actually see the movement of *prana,* as it is called in India, or *chi,* as it is called in China. You can feel it radiating from all forms of life in nature, from people, and even from so-called inanimate objects that have power, such as art or sculpture that was created with intention.

Intention is a key word here. Intention combined with attention creates opportunity to make something happen, to harness and direct energy to manifest in specific ways, for specific purposes. In the work of Alchemical Healing, intention and attention are keys that unlock the mystery of healing, of co-creating reality, and of manifesting your most fulfilling destiny.

Physical health is directly related to energy, whether it is energy that heals or energy that stops you cold in your tracks. Dealing with energy is the crux of the matter. The exercises in this book will help you develop your focus and your powers of attention and concen-tration. And they will increase your sensitivity to all types of energy.

The more you pay attention to energy, the more aware you become of its subtler aspects. Often in this kind of healing work, less is more: the subtlest energies can make the greatest difference. The primary energy in Alchemical Healing is what we call the Universal Life Force—the infinite activity, the movements of light and vibratory frequencies that are the basic constituents of life. By whatever name it is called, and there are many, this life force energy can be channeled through your body in a way that regenerates you while you are simultaneously directing it out to others or into yourself with intention. This force is activated by intention, and it becomes more accessible through the attunements offered here.

When you have activated this energy within your own body system, you are connected to the infinite source and can now access it more strongly at will. There are many pathways and disciplines through which you can facilitate this connection. Alchemical Healing offers its own unique approach, through specific initiatory processes. Once the connection is made, you will have it for the rest of your life. Because the source is limitless, it will always be there. You cannot use it up, but keep in mind that you must stay aware of the difference between your personal store of energy and the infinite Universal Life Force.

One of the main pitfalls in healing is thinking that you are the one doing the healing. Therein lies the first paradox. *You are, and you are not.* You are the conduit through which the energy flows. There is an important distinction to make between your personal power and the Universal Life Force. If the power comes from you—from your personal store of energy—you have only a finite amount and can use it up, leaving yourself drained and vulnerable. If it comes *through* you, and you honor the infinite and intelligent source, then it will always be there for the asking, and it will never run out.

In our practice, the first attunement to access the Universal Life Force for doing healing work is called the Fire Mist Shower.

9
ACCESSING THE
UNIVERSAL LIFE FORCE

THE FIRE MIST SHOWER

The fire mist shower is an outpouring of energy that flows up your spine and out from the top of your head through your crown chakra, creating a fountain that showers over and around you. It is the primary current that we use for healing. When the current is flowing freely without blockages, it purifies, invigorates, and renews. You can extend it to shower over and around the person with whom you are working to create a space that is cleansed and protected as well as an energetic connection between you. This outpouring of life force energy, or prana, can be directed to come through your hands and fingertips at will. The initiation you are about to receive will activate this shower and provide you with a trigger mechanism for instant access to this energy.

Additionally, this attunement opens the eyes in the palms of your hands, providing an extrasensory perception that is important to the intuitive assessments required during the process of Alchemical Healing. The third eye and the eyes in the palms of your hands are etheric organs of sensitivity that, although they don't appear in our

Western anatomy books, are referred to in many Eastern texts. You will find them prevalent in the spiritual art of India, Tibet, and even in the art of the northwest Native American tribes of the United States and Canada. Later in this chapter we will cover the development of the actual sense perception of these eyes.

First you must decide upon a word of intrinsic power, which you will use to invoke this potent energy force. The word that you choose will not only be the trigger, it will also automatically imbue the process for which it is used with the qualities it represents. It also focuses your attention, stops you from merely acting as though you are doing something, and creates a *fait accompli*. For example, if you choose the word *light*—or *compassion,* or *love*—every time you use that word with intention, the energy will immediately turn on and whatever you do next will be invested with additional light or compassion or love. If you choose a word that we use commonly in conversation, it will only affect you in this special way when you use it with intention, not at other times when used causally. Also, it is important to keep your magical connection with this word sacred, and it is therefore best not to speak of it to others.

If you choose the name of a deity for your word, such as Isis or Kuan Yin, take a moment to tune in first to ask permission of that being, because every time you use the word you will be connecting directly with the energy of that deity. Do the same if you wish to use a power animal or plant spirit for this connection. In choosing the best word, consider your aspirations. What attribute would you most like to add to your healing powers? If you choose a word with no intrinsic value or meaning, it will still work as the trigger mechanism that shifts your reality and turns the flow of energy on.

The word that you use as your power word should be kept private. Continue working with it until you have absorbed its power and this power has become part of you. Then, if you feel the need, you can reinitiate yourself to a new word with different attributes.

If you cannot think of an appropriate word, take the time you need to journey to Thoth, or another appropriate ally, to request suggestions. I have been using the same word for more than twenty years. When it was first given to me, I did not fully understand its meaning. Although it took me years to grow into it, it has always brought power and energy into my work.

This initiation can be taken by anyone, as each person will open to the process to the degree of his or her individual preparedness. Every person who follows these instructions will be able to access the infinite Universal Life Force for healing and will be able to learn the various ways it can be used as shown throughout this book. Those who wish to attain deeper levels of this initiation can seek assistance from an authorized Alchemical Healing instructor.

I suggest that you read the text of this initiation once before you actually engage in the practice. If you are working with another person or in an alchemical study group, it may be helpful to have your partner read aloud to you while you perform the visualization. Or you may want to record your own voice reading the instructions. It is also important to maintain focus and intention on the goals of this attunement as you move through the process, especially when it comes time to repeat your word.

THE EFFECTS OF THE FIRE MIST SHOWER
- Accesses the Universal Life Force
- Enhances the clairvoyant abilities of the third eye
- Opens the eyes in the palms of your hands
- Opens the circuits to the palms of the hands and fingertips through which energy is generated
- Cleanses and invigorates the chakras
- Creates a protective energy field

PREPARATION
During the first activation of the Fire Mist Shower you will be given specific openings that you need only receive once in this lifetime. This initiation is a major adjustment and needs to be treated with respect. Once the initial openings are in place, subsequent practice

of the Fire Mist Shower as a meditation (without the initial activating process) will be integral to the practice of Alchemical Healing, and will be described following the initiation.

Prepare an appropriately sacred space to conduct this ritual. Do whatever is comfortable to enhance the moment—build an altar, light a candle, smudge the space or light incense.

INITIATION

ACTIVATING THE FIRE MIST SHOWER

Begin by choosing your word, as described above.

Sit up as straight as you can, with your spinal column perpendicular to the floor or chair or ground. (If that is impossible for you, look within and visualize yourself sitting cross-legged with your back straight, and work within that image.)

Ground and center, using the breath to fill your belly on the inhale, and then exhale downward, through your tailbone to connect yourself with the earth. . . .

Devote attention to your heart flame, directing love to make it grow and spread its radiance throughout your being, filling you with warmth and light. . . .

Stir the waters within your golden cauldron. Notice as the waters rise to meet the flame in your heart, and experience the conversion as the water meets the fire and turns to steam. . . .

The steam rises, opening the shamanic passageway at your throat and filling your head. Place your entire attention within the steam. As it gathers in your head, it will lift your consciousness up through your crown and into your light body. . . .

Thoth comes from the left to greet you. He will be there to witness and assist as needed in this process. He will also record this activity in the book of your soul's life.

Establish your connection with Thoth. . . .

Begin to extend your attention deep into the earth. Notice as you travel downward, layer by layer, an increase in warmth and fluidity as you move toward the core. There is an orange glow. . . .

You will know when you have arrived at the source of energetic nourishment at the heart of the earth. . . .

Begin to draw that energy back up, opening a channel that will always be there for you. . . . The energy rises up through this channel and begins to move from your tailbone at the root chakra, up through your body. . . .

Feel it energize and set each chakra to spinning in turn. . . . As the current of energy rises inside of you, the power floods upward through your body, awakening, revitalizing, purifying, renewing. . . .

Pay special attention when the current reaches and mingles with the fire in your heart. . . . Then let it continue up until it reaches your third eye. . . .

Take the necessary time to let the current work its way upward. . . . When the flow of energy reaches your third eye, stop and allow the energy to collect there. . . .

Begin repeating your chosen word to yourself, silently, seven times—one for each of seven breaths. As you repeat your word the energy that has been rising within you becomes very concentrated at your third eye, cleansing and awakening this center to the degree that your system can handle at this time. . . .

After seven breaths with seven repetitions of your word, the energy is now free to continue up to the top of your head and on out through your crown like a fountain, making the Fire Mist Shower. . . .

Take a few moments to feel this constant stream of energy as it continues to flow up through your body and out through your crown. The current may start as a small trickle that will grow as you continue to focus your attention upon it. The fountain also grows with use, until you are able to control it somewhat, even to direct its power so that you can extend it to cover considerable space surrounding you. Stay with this visualization and the vital feeling of this fountain shower until you have reached and can maintain a sense of fullness. This will be different for each person. You can recognize it as the moment when the growth of the current and fountain stops—remaining steady without further expansion. . . .

This first time, when the energy is moving freely and as you continue to feel the flow moving up and out of your crown, bring your attention to your hands and point them, palms extended, toward Thoth, who has been observing and assisting throughout this process. With a deft motion, he opens the energy centers in the eyes in the palms of your hands. You will feel an opening as the current begins to flow out of them. Feel the energy flowing out like great rays of light emanating from your palms. . . .

Next Thoth will touch each of your fingertips, releasing the energy so that beams of light can radiate from the newly opened tips of your fingers. . . .

Linger in this space, feeling the energy flow grow and regulate itself until you feel solid and complete with this experience. . . .

Take time to listen for any message Thoth may have for you at this moment regarding this initiation and your healing work. He could have some very specific instructions for you. . . .

Before you open your eyes, and while the first flow of energy is still strong in your hands and fingertips, direct the energy to someone you know who is in need of healing. Use your newly awakened third eye to perceive the person in whatever way he or she comes to you. Do not be attached to seeing visually; feel free to use your imagination or memory to conjure up the person you have chosen. . . .

Now visualize the person as being already healed. See him as you know he can be, dancing and singing in the universe, or in whatever situation best expresses to you that person's most vital potential for health. . . .

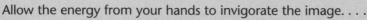

Allow the energy from your hands to invigorate the image. . . .

When the thought form that you have created feels full and complete, release the image and blow on your open hands to break the connection. Immediately the current will stop flowing from your hands, or at least subside considerably.

Take a moment to feel yourself whole and unattached, yet still filled with light and surrounded by the Fire Mist Shower. . . .

Express your gratitude to Thoth and receive his blessing and any further messages or instructions he has for you at this time. . . .

Ground and center yourself. When you are ready, open your eyes.

Take a few moments to rest in the connection that now exists, then close your eyes and repeat your word to yourself once again, silently. Notice that the Fire Mist Shower starts up immediately, and that if you desire to do healing work, the energy is there instantly, pouring from your hands.

PRACTICING THE FIRE MIST SHOWER

The Fire Mist Shower can be practiced as a meditation to awaken and cleanse your chakras and energy conduits each morning, or at any time during the day. To use it as a meditation, simply ground and center yourself and take a moment to quiet your mind. Use your power word with the intention of engaging your Fire Mist Shower. Focus your attention on the energy that moves up your body and out through your crown, paying special attention when it passes up through your heart and mingles with your heart flame. Use your word with intention to release the current of energy and bring it up and out through your crown and your hands. Let it flow and bask in the light of your Fire Mist Shower. Allow yourself to feel the cleansing and regeneration it provides.

I use my Fire Mist Shower at the beginning of each healing session, as well as any time that I personally need a boost in energy. It can be instigated quite quickly, instantly actually, by saying your word with intention and focus. At times that require special attention, I will use my word like a mantra, repeating it over and over to merge the power and energy of this initiation into whatever work I am doing. As you continue to use this powerful tool, you will find that it becomes an intrinsic part of your approach not only to healing, but to all creative aspects of your life.

It should be noted that although the Fire Mist Shower is generated from deep in the earth, the Universal Life Force itself actually comes from a different source, one whose activation is part of the mystery of the initiation.

GENERATING THE ENERGY FOR HEALING

We will devote the rest of this chapter to some exploratory exercises to help you become more comfortable with the healing energy and to get a sense of the different ways it works. Now that you have accessed the Universal Life Force, you can begin to use it for healing. It will always be available to you. It is activated by your intention to heal and boosted by your word and its intrinsic qualities. It can also be stimulated by need, such as when you pass an accident on the highway. Or, if you walk through a corridor in a hospital and put your palms out, you may notice that there is a surge as you pass each door.

It would be beneficial to gain experience by working on a real pain or problem as soon as you have the opportunity. If available, you can work on a friend or even a pet or house plant for practice. It will be a stronger experience for you if there is a specific problem to address. The place of need in a person's body will recognize the energy source that you have become, and will automatically begin to draw on that energy when you direct your hands toward the problem with intention.

To reiterate, it is important to realize that the energy you are sending is not coming from your personal supply. Remember, through this initiation you have been connected with an infinite source, and if you use it consciously, your personal energy will not be depleted.

Sometimes, when I am very tired—so tired that I can't imagine doing anything—I am called upon to do the Work. Occasionally, I can barely manage to lift my hands and aim them toward the person, whether they are right in front of me or at a distance.

First of all, you should remember to take care of yourself and not let yourself get so tired. But if you do find yourself in such a state, and you need to practice healing, you will quite likely find that the Work will regenerate you and give you the boost that is needed to accomplish whatever challenge is before you. There is, however, a point of diminishing returns. You can stay more focused and direct the healing better if you are not exhausted.

Another question that needs to be addressed is this: When is it not appropriate for a person to direct healing toward others? Certainly there might be occasions when you are sick or weak. Sometimes you simply get the message that this work is not for you to do at this time, or for this person. It is always your option and right to decide not to practice healing in any given situation. This subject is further developed in the ethics chapter.

Some people have a tendency to think that they are not good enough or healthy enough to perform this work. It's true that you can spend a lifetime healing and perfecting yourself. That is a job that is never complete, however, and if you wait until you think you are close enough to perfect, you will never extend your healing powers toward others.

In my experience, it was through doing the healing work that I received the most healing. As my healing practice escalated, I noticed that my habits naturally became healthier. I became more sensitive and recognized the effect different substances had on my life and on those around me. My desire to facilitate healing in others resulted in my own healing, because as the energy passed through my system, it left a bit of itself with me.

EXERCISE
Transmitting the Energy

The purpose of this exercise is to get the feel of how the healing energy works, how you turn it on and off, and what it feels like to give energy and receive it. It is most helpful to have a friend with whom you can practice and communicate the experience and results. If your friend is also learning from this book and has taken the Fire Mist Shower initiation, you can take turns. If you don't have someone to work with, try working on a pet or a plant, even though you won't have the benefit of a verbal response.

Start by determining where on the person's body you wish to apply the energy. If possible, choose a place that is in need, because need acts like a sponge that recognizes the source of energy and draws upon it. This will make the feeling of the transmission of energy more palpable. If the person is healthy and has no specific pain, go for the shoulders. Almost all of us carry stress in our shoulders.

Ground and center yourself, and use your word to create the Fire Mist Shower while setting your intention to transmit the Universal Life Force for healing. . . .

Place your hands directly on the body part, keeping your hands still and your fingers close together. Usually, just seconds after your intention is set and you've said your word silently, there is a response that feels as though a tap has been turned on in the ethers, and there is a surge as the current rushes through you and flows from your hands, entering the place of your focus.

This energy can feel hot or cool, tingly or electric, or it can simply be a vibration or frequency that you will learn to recognize with practice. And the feeling will change from time to time. The initiation of the Fire Mist Shower has opened the eyes of perception that exist in the palms of your hands. As you begin to learn the language of these eyes in your palms, you will be able to interpret for yourself what is happening with the energy at any given moment.

Even during your first experiment, you may be able to feel that initial surge as the energy flows into the place where your focus is. After a while the current will begin to ebb, and you will know that the chosen place has received all it needs for the time being. Do not feel distraught if you cannot feel the energy the first time you try. You are working with subtle levels of reality, and it sometimes takes time and practice to awaken your sensitivities. . . .

Next try to transmit the energy into the first auric field of your partner. The aura is the energetic field that surrounds a living organism. It is like the glow around a candle flame, although more subtle, and it can be seen by sensitive individuals as a transparent aureole that changes hues. To find this first auric field, start by turning on the energy with intention; then open your hands to feel the energetic field at some distance from the body, approximately two feet. Slowly bring your hands closer in toward the body and feel for any changes in the field. At approximately three to eight inches, give or take a few, you will feel a subtle resistance. This is the area of the first auric field. Using your intention, and saying your word to yourself, repeat the exercise as you did a moment ago, but now work with your hands at this small distance from your partner's body. Once again you will feel the surge as the power is turned on and the energy moves through you. Allow it to pour through you until it ebbs. Pay close attention to the feelings, especially in the palms of your hands and your fingertips. . . .

Often the light coming off your palms and fingertips naturally ebbs as you complete your work. If it continues, or is uncomfortable, simply blow on your hands with the intention of discontinuing the flow, and pass your palms across each other, and it will stop.

We are like straws that get coated with the milk that passes through them. We are the recipients of the life force energy every time we turn our hands toward healing. So in a very real way, every time we attempt to heal another, we are also healing ourselves.

Directing energy with "hands on" (meaning hands physically touching the body) and healing through the auric field are both viable techniques, and each has its time and place. For some people it is very important to receive hands-on healing, simply for the touch. Many people who need healing are also in need of being touched in a loving way. Often the energies are turned on in conjunction with massage or other healing work that requires touch, such as acupressure or even acupuncture.

There are many theories about the auric fields, as to how many there might be and what each one holds. For our purposes, it is only important to note that an auric field extends from the body and is varyingly accentuated for some distance before it becomes inextricably connected with the fields of everything else in creation.

The construction of a building must conform to its blueprint in order to maintain integrity. The first auric field is like the blueprint of the body. In healing it functions the same way: if you change the basic plan of the blueprint, the physical body will change to conform to the blueprint. Working in the auric field accesses energies and patterns of health or disease before they actually happen in the physical body. To a proficient medical intuitive, cancer, for example, will be recognizable in the field before it has actually taken hold in the physical body.

My personal preference is to work in the auric field, so I do most of my healing work without actually touching the body of the recipient. I find the auric field stronger, and I can feel without the distraction of touch what the eyes in my hands are telling me.

SEEING WITH THE EYES IN THE HANDS

One of the advantages of receiving access to the Universal Life Force through the Fire Mist Shower initiation is the opening of the eyes in the palms of your hands. Not only is the volume and quality of accessible energy enhanced, but the renewal of the ability to *see* through your hands, which has been lost to most of us, brings another informative dimension to the healing work.

You have probably seen Tibetan, East Indian, and northwest Native American art that portrays characters with eyes painted on their foreheads, the palms of their hands, and the soles of their feet. These pictorial representations depict sensitivities that, though acknowledged as natural by some cultures, are given no credence in our own. Because of our lack of identification with these metaphysical organs of sensitivity, we must learn to utilize them in much the same way we learn a new language.

When the eyes in the palms of our hands are open, they perceive through interaction with energy and can inform us in a variety of ways, according to our own method of accessing information beyond the physical realm. When some people turn their hands toward a person, a part of the body, or even a situation, it can be like turning on a movie projector. There are those who see in swift glimpses, whereas others hear, feel, or simply know. Our perception may, or may not, resemble the way we access information in our journey work.

Here is where you may discover special gifts that you may not have known you possessed, for example, the ability to *see* and/or *know* what is happening inside a person. While you hold your hands over an afflicted area, be open to any intuitive flashes that come *before* you begin to think about it. For many of us, intuition flies by without notice, because it happens so fast. It is easy to be distracted by thoughts about how things could or should be and miss that first intuitive knowing. If you find yourself trying to figure it out, you've already missed it. But don't despair; you have many ways to inform yourself, and all of them can be developed with practice.

For me, seeing with my hands is not visual; it comes through feelings. An entirely new kinesthetic language arose in me after the eyes in my palms were first opened, and it took considerable time and practice for me to learn, and gain confidence in, this new language, so that I could understand what my hands were telling me. The feelings seemed quite faint and undefinable as I began to explore and tried to distinguish them from one another. Gradually, as the sensations became more distinct, I recognized subtle differences and patterns of feeling that, through repetition, took on clear meaning. Even now, after years and years of practice, I still experience new feelings and subtle nuances that help me to know what is going on at any given moment during a healing.

As you become comfortable with directing energy through your hands, you will find a clear distinction between the times when the energy is flowing and when it is not. Associated feelings might include temperature differentials, tingling, vibrations, a sense of electricity or magnetism, a feeling of current or flow, tugging sensations, and other signals. It is not necessary to be able to put into words the ways in which you experience the energy flow. Your relationship with the energy is a personal one, and although others may be able to describe theirs, it may not be perceived by you in quite the same way. In the beginning, it is sometimes confusing or intimidating to compare experiences unless we remember that each of our own unique ways of experiencing the flow is precious and valid.

As I continued to develop my healing work through practice, I found it easier to interpret the different sensations in my hands. Warmth might indicate that there is activity or inflammation. A cool breeze might suggest a tear or opening from which energy is escaping.

For me the energy felt as though I was plugged into a wall socket, with a current of electricity moving through my hands with varying strength, depending on the need of the individual I was working on. That information became quite useful in determining where to place my hands over the body. If I scanned the body from several inches above the surface of the skin, as though my hand were a metal detector, I could sense the need from a particular place as I passed over it. It was as though my hands provided a source of energy and the needy place in the body recognized the proximity of the source and drew from it. The stronger the need, the stronger the draw.

Sometimes I experience the connection as a particular twinge, or a kind of drag or catch on the energy, right in the palm of my hand. The precise nature of the feeling often tells me what I am connecting to. For instance, a very high-pitched frequency may identify a nerve, whereas a lower tone could define a bone or organ. These sensations are difficult to categorize because each person—having his own feelings—can only determine what they mean with time and practice.

What you *can* know is that certain feelings that you have will become consistent and many will also be felt by the person you are working on. For example, if you make a direct connection with a source of pain and *feel* it with the eyes in your hands, there is a very good chance that the person you are working on will feel what you are feeling as well. Ask her. Once you have made that connection and start to draw the energy of the pain out of the body, if you are successful, you may notice a twinge that feels as though something energetic is actually hitting the palm of your hand as it is released from the person's body. That release can be felt by the person whose pain is leaving. Again, remember to ask her. Be sure the person remains attentive to the place on which you are working.

Here there is a phenomenon that is still a mystery to me: those people who have the sensitivity to feel the process are more likely to have positive results than those who are unable to experience the work. That does not mean that the healing won't have results if a person doesn't feel it; however, the effectiveness is often greater when she does. Why some people are more sensitive than others is a curious thing. It has been my observation that different variables, such as the ability to focus and the level of skepticism, affect sensitivity. Sometimes it is just a mystery. I do believe that practicing the Fire Mist Shower and having the eyes in the palms of one's hands open increases the sensitivity to receive.

I have learned to rely quite heavily on my own sensitivities. If I am working on someone and I feel the connection and perhaps the subsequent release of pain or the spirit of the disease, I *know* that something has occurred. Sometimes I *know* that a healing has achieved the removal of the illness or pain or that there has been a harmonizing of the person's body. With pain, it is easy to get corroboration—the pain is either there or it is not. Or it can be more or less intense. When dealing with something like the removal of a tumor, the healing is less obvious, unless the tumor was protruding and the physical protrusion disappears. Although that has been known to happen, usually it takes some time between when the spirit of the growth or tumor is removed and the physical dissolution occurs. Even when you've come to rely on your own sensitivities, corroboration with a physician concerning measurable ailments is very helpful, and if you are working with something dangerous I would always recommend that you double-check your work with a medical professional.

Another feeling to look for is the sense of pulling that occurs when you use your hand like a magnet to pull out pain and other things. To help the person connect to the experience, you might tell her to pay close attention and look for that magnetic feeling. Or the feeling of suction like a vacuum cleaner. Energy release often feels as though an actual magnet is pulling iron filings from sand.

Even if you are a nonseer, you can translate images into feelings. It is also important to note that the images used do not have to be anatomically correct. I remember the first time I connected knowingly to a nerve: it *felt* as though it was a corroded battery cable. Regardless of the imaginative picture that might create, it was the appropriate image for the moment, and I was able to apply my skill blending the intuitive with the practical to inspire a course of action. Often the feelings you receive manifest in metaphors. And any metaphor that is effective is appropriate. What is important is to learn through practice how information comes to you. It can come like the images in an anatomy book, or like a cartoon, or through feelings that reveal their meanings through repetition. Over time, you will make more sense of your experience if you continue to work with it.

GIVING AND RECEIVING

My left hand is receptive and my right hand generative. If you haven't noticed the natural inclination of your own hands, I suggest you use the left to pull and the right to transmit, because that is the way it works for most people. I try to stay ambidextrous by alternating from time to time, but it is always a good idea to work with the natural direction of things. Each person must experiment and work this out for himself.

I like to scan for information with my left hand and generate with my right. I make all my laser incisions for psychic surgery with my right hand, with my fingertips. Most often, I start each healing by generating the life force from both hands and scanning the situation to get a sense of what is needed. I start out looking for information by running my left hand over the person's body, or the area in need of healing. I usually keep my hand at the level of the first auric field.

When I am clearly connected I like to communicate with my client. I learn a lot about his sensitivity to this work from the very beginning through dialogue, because most often he will feel the connection as soon as I do, especially if I call his attention to it. This also allows him to participate in his own healing.

Often I will pull or tug gently, usually with my left hand, pulling out as if my hand were a magnet, feeling for a certain sense of connection to the source of the problem. My intention is to make contact with the spirit of the disease, trauma, or pain. I feel that connection as movement or as a twinge that tells me something is there. Then I begin to draw out, pulling into my hand, feeling for the release as the spirit yields itself to me. When releases occur, I follow the all-important step of conducting the energies and offering them to Mother Earth for transformation into their highest potential.

Communication during this process is especially useful for novices who are learning to understand and interpret their feelings. When contact is made, and particularly when there is any release, an attentive patient will feel the release at the same moment you do. After you have established precedent, the signals are obvious. I imagine that it is similar to learning to feel the different pulses that are found in the wrist when practicing Chinese medicine. To the unschooled person, the differences are very subtle; but if you are trained, they are obvious.

Often the source of the pain will move, as if trying to run away. This happens frequently with a headache. When it starts to move, it is easy to track it and pull it out. It is also very important to refill with Universal Life Force each cavity from which you have drawn energy. (This is one of the four rules of Alchemical Healing, on which I will elaborate in Chapter 12.)

The following is an exercise that you can practice with someone else to experience what it feels like, and looks like, to see into another person's body.

EXERCISE
Developing X-Ray Vision

The purpose of this exercise is to learn to use the eyes in your hands to retrieve information from inside another body. Take as much time as you need with each step.

Close your eyes, ground and center yourself. . . .

Place your hands on a friend, one on each forearm. Keep your fingers close together so that you can maintain a tight range of focus.

Generate your Fire Mist Shower and say your word with the intention of using the eyes in the palms of your hands. (You may find that your fingertips are especially sensitive and that you can retrieve information from them as well.)

As soon as you feel yourself link with the other person, direct your attention to the surface upon which your hands are resting. Hold your hands absolutely still and feel the texture of the fabric or skin beneath your hands. If it is fabric, examine the texture of it—its thickness, color, weave, wrinkles—without looking at or moving your hands. Notice how much information you can perceive using the eyes in your palms. . . .

Extend your consciousness to the area beneath the fabric, and focus your attention on the skin, noticing all that you can about the skin, its pores, its rhythms, its tone.

Extend your consciousness to the layer just under the surface of the skin. What is happening here? Can you perceive the capillaries, the fatty tissue? Is there movement? What colors do you see or feel?

Extend your consciousness deeper into the body. Can you find a blood vessel? Can you examine its walls? Do you feel the flow of the blood through the vessel? Can you sense the pulse of the flow of blood?

Go even deeper, find a strata of muscle. Is it rough or smooth, tense or relaxed, hard or soft?

And again, go deeper still, until you reach the surface of bone. Is it wet or dry? Rough or smooth? Brittle or pliant? What color is it?

Now direct your consciousness into the center of the bone, to the place where the marrow resides and the red blood cells are being manufactured. . . . What information is here? Is there any activity? Sound? Movement?

From your heart, request the attention of the spirit of the bone, or of the entire skeletal system. As you call forth this spirit, hold the intention of wanting to be given a message from the spirit of bone about the health and needs of the bones of the person.

Do not be attached to the way the spirit presents itself. It could come in a way that is anatomically correct, or it could come as a comic strip character, or in unique symbols that are personally relevant. Simply allow yourself to accept the information, and experience it as it comes, and have a dialogue with the spirit in whatever way is easiest. . . .

Thank the spirit for responding.

And finally, very slowly, begin to withdraw your focus, layer by layer, gently removing yourself from the recipient's body until you find yourself back in your own body once again. Disconnect completely with your intention. If you feel the need, you can brush the surface of your hands together to break the connection.

Share any messages and insights you received and bring sacred closure to the experience. . . .

Remember, it is the *process* that is most important. When we are invested in a specific outcome, we tend to sabotage ourselves and our experience. When we stay present to the process, we find ourselves fully available to whatever information we are given at the moment.

10
THE ELEMENTS

LEARNING ABOUT THE ELEMENTS

The Universal Life Force is the primary energy that automatically springs from your hands and fingertips when you practice Alchemical Healing. When you understand and use the *elements,* you augment this energy with distinctive powers that can add to your precision and effectiveness.

To know the elements is to know ourselves and to have a greater understanding of the natural world around us. It appears as though our modern Western civilization, in its ongoing attempts to conquer nature, has separated itself from the elements and thus lost its vital contact with much of the essence of life. Spiritual and mystical traditions ponder the fundamental nature of reality; many honor the basic elements in their rituals and practices. The Western magical traditions of Europe and Native America incorporate four elements into their belief systems. In India the four elements derive from a matrix of ether or spirit. In China there is a five-element system, which includes metal and wood.

Each system provides a window into how our reality is molded. Working knowledge of any of these systems is useful, because the basis of alchemy is the mixing of elements to create transformation for an intended goal of healing or enlightenment.

Alchemical Healing uses five elements: *Earth, Water, Fire, Air,* and *Akasha. Earth* is substantive, relating to physicality and matter. *Water* flows, is wet and reflective, and is associated with the feminine. *Fire* is masculine, relates to energy, and is dry and active. *Air* is mental and associated with sound and communication. *Akasha* is the matrix from which the other four elements are derived, and is a universal solvent. There is a sweet simplicity to working with the individual components rather than being buried under the barrage of the totality of all creation.

Each element has its own dimension or realm and is associated with a chakra center, a symbol, and in some systems, other correspondences. We use the symbols that are associated with each element to create doorways through which we access each element for healing. Once accessed, each element can be directed in its pure energetic form through the hands and fingers of the initiate.

To learn about your personal proclivities toward one or more of the elements, it can be helpful to consult an astrologer. Our planets are in specific signs, each corresponding to elements, which in turn give us more detailed information about ourselves. I have a number of planets in the Air sign Gemini, as is obvious to those who have the knack for reading people elementally. Gemini is ruled by Mercury, which is associated with Thoth. I tend to move quickly and often, both physically and conversationally, and my gifts are very strong in communication and other functions associated with the element Air.

When you are aware of the unique intelligence inherent in the elements, you can use their specific energetic power in Alchemical Healing. You can enter the realms of the elements, known by some traditions as the elemental kingdoms, and interact directly, or invoke their spirits into your magical rituals. These spirits or elemental denizens are the fairies (Air), undines and mermaids (Water), elves and gnomes (Earth), and salamanders (Fire), all of whom most purely represent the elements themselves. Each expresses the nature, feelings, meaning, and intelligence in distinctive ways unique to that element. To put it another way, each element has spirit, spiritual intelligence, and a domain within which these can be encountered.

We can travel directly into the elemental realms and relate directly to the elemental beings, from whom we can learn a great deal about the elements themselves.

When we work with elements in Alchemical Healing, we are working with the *energy* of the elements rather than the elemental beings. That way, we are directing the essence of the element and can determine precisely which attributes or qualities we are drawing upon, as is appropriate to the moment.

For instance, to heal a laceration requires the buildup of new cells, actual physical material that forms to close and seal the cut. The element best suited for this task would be Earth, because it is the primary element of matter. If the laceration is infected, I would also use the element Water, because water can help to cleanse and cool the area.

Following are some exercises designed to help you create and maintain relationships with the elements.

EXERCISES
The Elements

Exercise One:

Take a pen and paper, and make yourself comfortable, preferably in a place of nature. Smudge yourself or purify in some way, then ground and center yourself. Open your heart to the space around you and ask for help in getting to know the elements. Put aside your notion of what you *think* they are. Sit quietly and notice how your senses perceive the elements. When you take a breath, what do you notice? Write down your perceptions. Go through each of the elements and describe what they are to you.

Exercise Two:

I highly recommend you journey with the lioness in *Power Animal Meditations,* because you will find clear and safe access into the elemental realms where you meet the inhabitants directly. Meanwhile, for this exercise, choose a specific element to meditate on. Picture yourself in a scene in your inner landscape where that element is prevalent. For example, if you have chosen Water, perhaps you will envision a special lake or stream, or ocean beach. Enter the water. Feel it. Move around in it. Perceive the water as you have always known it to be. Now put out your wishes to go beyond. See who comes to you to introduce you to the element Water. This being is part of the energy of Water.

This exercise is designed to help you connect with images from the deep well of your unconscious, and to become comfortable with being able to see and interpret from a new and expanded perspective. By exploring each element in this way, you accumulate a context within which to understand the energies of the elements.

Exercise Three:

Children have a more acute way of experiencing elements than adults. Meditating to remember childhood experiences in the natural world can help you gain direct access into the elements. Take a moment to remember yourself as a child and use a favorite memory as a key to unlock the doors into the elements. Acknowledge the wild abandonment of childhood, when you were first discovering the world around you and everything was new. If you loved to climb trees, remember your favorite tree, climb it, and from that place remember your relationship to the elements. From the perspective of your child self, remembering ocean swims and lake dips, climbs across great boulders (or even brick walls), campfire gazing, or explorations of caves will also help to invoke the elements.

With an understanding of the elements comes the ability to see people in terms of their elemental make-up. Their behavior and body language give clues as to how the elements are balanced within them. That information will help you to know when to add and when to remove elements in your healing work.

When you are directing energy for healing you can direct specific elements for specific purposes. For example, Water would be used to cool burns and cleanse or flush the body of toxins, and Earth would be used to help mend broken bones. The more information and experience you have about the elements, the more precise you can be in using them.

SYMBOLS

In Alchemical Healing, *symbols* are the tools we use to gain access to the elements. We live in a rich, multidimensional reality. Many unseen layers are combined to create the three-dimensional physical world that we perceive with our senses. Symbols provide access into these hidden worlds; they span the gaps between dimensions.

To have direct access to the elements in this system requires an initiation or adjustment within which your hands are rewired so that each finger is connected with a specific element. Symbols are used to create windows through which to access each element. Once initiated, you will simply draw the appropriate symbol in the air with the finger that is associated with that element, and that particular elemental domain becomes open, allowing the pure energy of the element to enter this realm. You can then direct that element through both your hands and all your fingertips, in the same way that you direct the Universal Life Force.

Each element has associations with all aspects of nature. As you begin to see things, people, and even situations elementally, a rich, enormous base of information appears, and the pure elemental energy that you can direct as a result of the rewiring is literally at your fingertips.

It is essential to know the attributes of the elements. The following descriptions of the elements include the symbols, fingers, and chakras associated with them in Alchemical Healing and some ideas about when to use them.

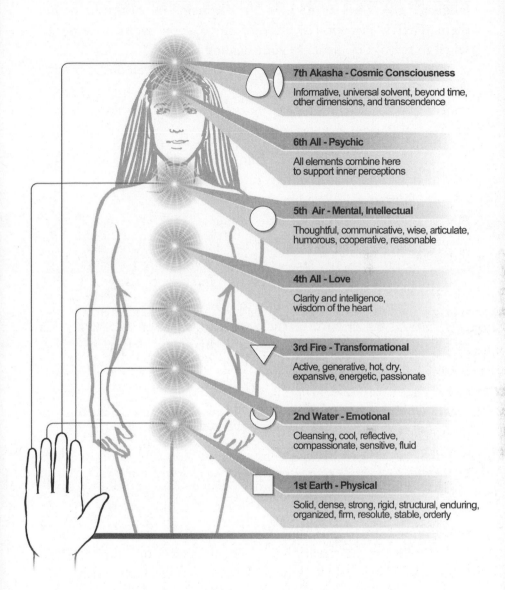

7th Akasha - Cosmic Consciousness

Informative, universal solvent, beyond time,
other dimensions, and transcendence

6th All - Psychic

All elements combine here
to support inner perceptions

5th Air - Mental, Intellectual

Thoughtful, communicative, wise, articulate,
humorous, cooperative, reasonable

4th All - Love

Clarity and intelligence,
wisdom of the heart

3rd Fire - Transformational

Active, generative, hot, dry,
expansive, energetic, passionate

2nd Water - Emotional

Cleansing, cool, reflective,
compassionate, sensitive, fluid

1st Earth - Physical

Solid, dense, strong, rigid, structural, enduring,
organized, firm, resolute, stable, orderly

***Figure* 10.1.** *The Elements Associated with Each Chakra*

THE FIVE-ELEMENT SYMBOL SYSTEM

EARTH

Nature—physical

Symbol—yellow square or cube

Ring finger (note that this is the stiffest or least flexible finger)

Chakra—first, root, base of spine

Characteristics—physical, solid, weighty, dense, strong, structural, manifestation into physical form, endurance and stamina, reliability, firmness, resolution—it contains and limits

- When Earth is balanced in a person, he or she is— stable, secure, strong, grounded, organized, considerate, honest, patient, objective, reliable, punctual, efficient, able to manifest needs
- Excess of Earth—stubborn, ultraconservative, rigid, stuck, unable to change, uptight, acquisitive, greedy, overindulgent
- Lack of Earth—unstable, lacking cohesion, weak, can't hold it together, unable to manifest
- Problems with Earth—stubborn, unscrupulous, insipid, dull, tardy, self-righteous, immobile

Earth is a combination of the other elements. It is solid and dense; it has weight and substance. It has form. It is the doorway through which all things come into being. We are born of Earth when we manifest in our bodies. Physical healing and manifestation of anything in physical form is done with the element Earth. It is used to mend broken bones and torn or lacerated tissue. You can direct it to build stable foundations and to rebuild body parts. It can be used to build up matter and to create etheric tools used for healing. Though these tools are fabricated with your intention and the element Earth, they are not fully formulated in the physical world. Earth is also used to create a stable, protected containment within which to conduct the more advanced alchemical techniques, such as grounding patterns in the body that are brought forward through time with Akasha.

WATER

Nature—emotional
Symbol—silver crescent moon
Thumb
Chakra—second, genitals, womb
Characteristics—cooling, contracting, moist, cleansing, compassionate, nurturing, sensitive, reflective, intuitive, fluid, serene, calming, empathic, passive

- When Water is balanced in a person, he or she is— flexible, adaptable, fluid, nurturing, giving, compassionate, intuitive, sensitive, and caring
- Excess of Water—hypersensitive, fearful or paranoid, secretive
- Lack of Water—insensitive, lacking intimacy, unable to flow, feeling heat, stuck
- Problems with Water—poor boundaries, addictions, apathy, laziness, indifference, shyness, and depression

The crescent moon symbol often appeared in ancient cultures as a symbol of feminine archetypes. It exemplifies the moon and also symbolizes the horns of the water buffalo, representing the horned Egyptian goddess, Hathor.

In Alchemical Healing, Water is used to flush, to cool, to dissolve, and to cleanse. Because its primary association is with emotions, Water is useful in any healing of our emotional body, and especially to reduce emotional anguish. Water is also used to calm things down and as a medium to carry the spirits of herbs when desired. Anytime you are working with toxins, you can use the element Water to flush the area or system. It is especially important to use when working with drug and alcohol addiction.

FIRE

Nature—spiritual, transformative
Symbol—down-pointed red triangle
Index finger
Chakra—third, solar plexus
Characteristics—hot, dry, expansive, destructive,
  passionate, energetic, consuming, and quick. It also
  relates to activity, enthusiasm, eagerness, courage,
  vitality, excitement, willpower, and daring.

  ◆ When Fire is balanced in a person, he or she is—
    self-motivated, responsive, energetic, witty,
    passionate
  ◆ Excess of Fire—angry, violent, hyperactive, raging,
    vengeful, erratic in behavior
  ◆ Lack of Fire—sluggish, slow, dull, without energy,
    cold
  ◆ Problems with Fire include—gluttony, jealousy,
    obsessive behavior, fanaticism, irritability and
    destructive behavior

For healing, Fire is used to generate energy, to vitalize and stimulate.
Fire is also used to cauterize, and occasionally to fight fire with fire,
as with arthritis. (Most inflammations would rather be cooled with
Water.) Fire is also used to warm and expand, and to dry.

In the advanced alchemical work, Fire is used to combust old patterns, to burn away the old to make way for the new. When the region
you are working with is not too fragile, direct fire to break down or
destroy, as in the alchemical process of calcination. Fire can also be
condensed into a fine, penetrating laser for use in psychic surgery.

AIR

Nature—mental, intellectual
Symbol—blue circle or sphere
Little finger (that is the lightest finger)
Chakra—fifth, throat

Characteristics—lightness and spaciousness, humor, pleasure, sound, community, cooperation, vocalizing, intelligence, joy, optimism, adaptability, beauty, reason

+ When Air is balanced in a person, he or she is— thoughtful, communicative, wise, quick, funny, articulate, clever
+ Excess of Air—egghead, totally in brain, gossipy, quarrelsome, loud, flighty, silly, arrogant
+ Lack of Air—vacuous, thoughtless, overly hungry, stupid, irrational, claustrophobic
+ Problems with Air—fickle, dishonest, dramatic, defiant, mentally unstable

Air is the lightest element, and you can use it to lighten things up. I send Air to folks when things get too serious and to enhance communications. Air helps with mental clarity and can be directed toward those with mental problems. It is important to direct air to lung problems and to places that need more spaciousness or opening as part of their healing. It is also useful for making protective cushions to surround and protect injuries while they are healing. We are all connected through the element Air.

AKASHA

Nature—universal intelligence, the matrix that the other elements come from

Symbol—purple-black egg flecked with gold or indigo, vesica piscus

Middle finger (the tallest finger)

Chakra—seventh, crown

Characteristics—informative, beyond space and time, wisdom and knowledge, etheric flux, out of body and visionary experience, transmutation, universal solvent

+ When Akasha is balanced in a person, he or she will be—in touch with the High Self, capable of retrieving information from the past and future,

able to communicate beyond three dimensions,
willing to serve and help others, able to travel out
of the body, able to heal through time
- Excess of Akasha—disorientated, comatose
- Lack of Akasha—disoriented, self-centered, having
a narrow point of view
- Problems with Akasha—escapism, living in a
dreamworld, incapable of recognizing the fullness
of being, religious fervor, spiritual arrogance

Akasha is the basic medium of creation. It contains all potential and
all information—the basic patterns of creation. It is associated with
the crown chakra, because the crown is the doorway to the superconscious mind, the collective higher intelligence.

In healing work, we use Akasha to dissolve old patterns and create new ones. We enter Akasha to get information and to find the
original causes of disease or destructive patterns. It should be
explained that one can enter Akasha in two ways, depending upon
the purpose. Using the symbol of the purple-black egg, as in the
Cauldron Alchemy, manifests potential in this plane. The entire universe conspires to create a nurturing environment for creativity, and
for the birth of the product of creativity. The egg is a universal symbol of the creative process; the purple-black color, often flecked with
gold, is like the night sky, spangled with stars. This egg often
appears as a symbol of the source of the creative process, as in the
Journey to Thoth in Chapter 5.

Another symbol for Akasha is the *vesica piscus,* or, more literally, vessel of the fish. It also translates as fish bladder. The most
famous rendering of this symbol is found in Glastonbury, England,
on the cover of the Chalice Well. The sacred geometric design
comes from the interaction of two circles, one symbolizing above,
the other below. When these two circles intersect one another, the ()
that is created in the center represents above and below coming
together as one, and the portal into that dimension is the vesica pis-

cus. I like to use this symbol when I am doing healing work that verges on dancing. I sometimes use both hands to create this symbol; at other times I draw the symbol with a hand or finger in a small and subtle way.

Akasha is the most powerful element to work with. A chapter is devoted to it in the advanced section of this book.

SELF-INITIATING INTO THE ELEMENTS FOR HEALING

The basic energy that we work with is the Universal Life Force. Just as the sun's rays separate into the spectrum of colors when put through a prism, so the Life Force displays its spectrum of elements to those who have learned through initiation to perceive these elemental energies. For optimum effectiveness within this system, your hands and fingers need to be connected with the symbols so you can access the elements directly. A strand of aka from each finger and thumb will be woven with a strand of aka from each of the elemental domains. The aka can be seen or felt, depending upon your individual style of perception.

This wiring of your hands is best done by a teacher from this lineage; however, you can start the work on your own and begin to feel the difference. The following self-initiation provides a good beginning. If it resonates, you can seek an Alchemical Healing teacher in your area to deepen the process.

The symbols serve as windows into the dimensional realms of each element. Once accessed, each element can be directed in its pure energetic form through the hands and fingers of the initiate.

I recommend that you study the following instructions; then do the initiation by yourself. Although it may seem complicated at first glance, it is really simple, and the results are obvious and profound.

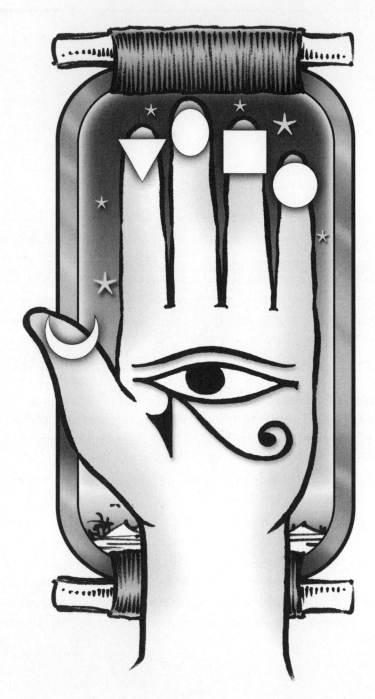

Figure 10.2. The Elements Associated with Each Finger by Symbol

INITIATION

CONNECTING TO THE ELEMENTS

Prepare as you would for a special journey. Ground and center yourself and use your power word to get the Fire Mist Shower flowing and the Universal Life Force moving through your hands. . . .

Set your intention to connect with the elements, starting with Water.

Draw the symbol of the element, in the case of Water the crescent moon with its points upturned, in the air with your thumbs, and you will create a window between this material plane and the elemental realm of Water. By putting both your hands into the window, thumbs first, you enter the dimension of Water. With the tips of your thumbs, reach for and grab hold of a piece of aka within the element. It will stick to your thumbs. Feel the fine, watery threads and pull them back through the window into this realm. Hold your hands up and open and feel the element as it moves from your thumb tips into the eyes in the centers of the palms of your hands. When you feel it connect in the centers of your palms, extend your hands back through the elemental window, thumb tips first, and with your intention, release a strand of your own personal aka out through your thumb tips and into the elemental realm. The process is very much like weaving spirit and elemental matter together, creating a living connection between your hands and the elements. When you bring your hands back through the window and into this plane, the rewiring of the thumbs with that specific element is complete, and you are ready to go on to the next element and next finger.

I suggest that you start with Water, and move on to Fire, Akasha, Earth, and Air, simply because of the order of the thumb and fingers. Use the forefinger, of course, when you are weaving

Fire, the middle finger for Akasha, and so on. Take a moment to feel the results after each element. You will notice very distinctive feelings. When all digits are connected, allow a few minutes to integrate the feelings, then blow on your hands and rub them together once or twice to break the connection.

HEALING WITH ELEMENTS

When you have completed the initiation and are ready to experience what you have accomplished, draw the elemental symbol of your choice with either or both of the appropriate fingers, put both your hands through the symbol, and let the energy flow from your hands toward your chosen recipient. The energy that is transmitted through your hands and all of your fingers will be quite specifically the element you have invoked. The initiation for connecting to the elements only needs to be done once, and the connection is made for this lifetime, although it does strengthen when you use the energy of the elements in your work. After you have self-initiated in this way, you can practice with a friend to get the sense of each element and how it feels to direct it. From this point forward, anytime you create the symbolic window with the appropriate finger, your hands will be transmitting that element in its pure energetic form as soon as you put them through the window.

When you work with the elements during healing, you can draw the symbol with one hand or two; you can draw it large or small. I generally draw it very small, so that I am not being obvious. Drawing it large would look quite weird at a restaurant, an airport, or a hospital—anyplace where I don't want to attract attention. There is no need to be dramatic or obvious when subtlety is sufficient. When I am giving private sessions or class demonstrations, especially while sharing certain advanced techniques with musical accompaniment, I sometimes become more animated and the movements become part of a healing dance.

When you transmit the elements during healing you do not need to move in the order listed above. You can move seamlessly from one element to another, depending on the need of the moment. If the energies feel as though they are not flowing, remember to boost things with your power word. Your intention is important here, as always. When you become proficient with using the elements in this way, it is very much like having a palette of colors to work with while creating a work of art. You can determine which element to use through your rational and practical mind, and you will also notice that when an element desires to be used, a fingertip might unaccountably twinge or quiver to get your attention. Always be aware of the signs that are occurring around you—nature and synchronicity often provide unexpected guidance. All intelligence is valid in this system.

It is important to honor your rational and practical mind, even while you function in the intuitive and mystical realms. As you come to understand the elements and their usefulness in healing, you will know when to use each one separately, and when they go together in sequence.

There is no need to sever the connection to one element before working with the next one when using the energy from your hands. It can be a fluid dance in which you are the choreographer with nature. The elements mix and blend in much the same way as colors. To get the best results, it is important to consider the ratio of each element to the other. Take Fire and Air as an example. Just enough air is fuel for fire, as with bellows, yet too much air will blow fire out, as with a candle. There are times to blend the elements, and times to use them as distinctly different tools that one might use one after the other.

A practice that you can do to deepen your perception of the elements is to imagine yourself sitting within the three-dimensional symbolic form of each of the four gross elements (Earth, Water, Fire, and Air). As you sit inside a yellow cube, or a blue sphere, and so on, you will feel yourself as if immersed in the element. Notice how it interacts with your body and psyche.

Now that you are hooked up with the elemental connection in your hands, you can have some fun. Try directing each element in turn and have the person you are working with guess which element you are using. The connection is always stronger if you are working on someone who is in need, but you should be able to feel the difference between the elements regardless. Play with temperature using Fire and Water. Improve someone's mood with Air.

When you are practicing Alchemical Healing, begin as usual with your connection, attention, and generation of the Universal Life Force using your power word. Insert the elements into your energetic transmissions as needed, allowing your knowledge of the elements and your intuition to guide you. Pay attention to each situation, and be willing to stretch yourself as you integrate these new tools.

EXAMPLES

Burns are a most obviously elemental condition, and the use of Water in treating them is the most obvious choice. Following are three examples of healing working with burns that utilized the element Water.

★ ☾ ★

As a result of removing the radiator cap prematurely from his overheated truck, Dan had second- and third-degree burns all over his chest. He spent four days in the hospital and had just returned home when I was asked to help him. I had never seen severe burns and was surprised at the depth of damage. It would have been impossible to lay hands directly on these deep wounds; there was no skin, and the dressings had to be changed two or three times a day. I could feel the heat generating from the burns, which seemed as though they were still burning, and Dan's continuing agony was apparent.

My intention was to somehow lessen the pain, plus I hoped I could stop the ongoing burning and begin to cool the area down. With those intentions I connected with my hands about six inches above Dan's chest. As the energy began to flow, I drew the symbol of Water and began to concentrate my attention on the cooling properties of water. Because of my schedule, I only had about twenty minutes to work on him, and then I was leaving town. Acutely aware of my time restrictions, I held my intention with strong focus as I continued pouring the energy of cool water into the burns, especially toward the deepest wounds. I clearly felt when the tide turned and the area began to cool. Some of the tension eased as the pain became more tolerable. It was the only session I was able to have with Dan, but as soon as he recovered he came for a visit and filled me in on what had happened. Although there was still pain after our session, it was far more manageable than the agony that had permeated him before my visit. From that point forward, the burns healed with great speed.

What most amazed the doctors who were working with Dan was that the deepest burns healed fastest, faster than the peripheral ones that I had not had time to work on. And there was no scarring.

★ ☾ ★

The following is from Danielle Hoffman, an Alchemical Healing instructor:

> My niece burned her hand on a hot stove when she was three and a half years old and was wailing in pain. I immediately drew the symbol for water and placed my hands over the burnt area. She stopped crying immediately and looked intensely at the space between our hands. I asked her if she could feel the cool water and she nodded her head yes. That's when I realized that she could see it as well as feel it. I asked her and she confirmed it with another nod of her head. After about two minutes she was fine. There were no blisters, and she went on with her playing and exploring.

The two things that amazed me the most about this impromptu healing were, first, that she stopped crying right away, and then, that she was intrigued with watching what was happening. The water not only soothed the burn, but also the emotions.

I had a friend who was an emergency room physician. He had an experience similar to Danielle's. One evening at the hospital a boy of about five was brought in. A pot of boiling water had fallen off the stove, and the boy was scalded and screaming in pain.

My friend wanted to do something to quiet the boy. He thought the Alchemical Healing work would do as well as anything else, so he asked the parent to wait for a moment outside the room. (He did this kind of work only in private at the hospital, to avoid confusing or disturbing people who did not understand what he was doing.) As soon as he called in Water and directed it onto the burns, the child stopped screaming. These burns were very severe, however, and though the child was no longer crying in agony, he still required treatment. My doctor friend did not follow up on his progress, but was very impressed with the initial reduction of pain. The pain did not recur during the time he was in the emergency room.

★ ☽ ★

Here is a brief, recent example involving the healing use of the element Air.

Morwen is a great drummer. She sees drumming in support of the magical fire/drum circles as a part of her service. We were at Firedance, a wonderful annual festival that we love to attend in Northern California. By the day after the first of four all-night fire circles, Morwen had already exacerbated the tendonitis and carpal tunnel syndrome she had been dealing with in her right elbow and thumb. Additionally, she had played the djembe, not her usual instrument, and the middle finger joint was inflamed.

When I connected up and checked in with her as I began the work, I asked her to tell me what she saw. Hawk appeared and gave her information about looking at the "big picture" in her visioning work. Taking my cue from Hawk, I realized that it was Air that would most help her, so that is what I used to create space and comfort around the inflamed area. I also used Water to cool the inflammation. Both I and another healer, Sylvia Brailer, worked on her that day and she finished the rest of the festival without any discomfort whatsoever.

I often use Air in this way to surround and protect internal areas that have been worked on, such as bone spurs and back injuries that require flexibility. When more stiffness is required, I build a splint with Earth.

As you explore the usefulness of the elements, be willing to ask for feedback from whomever you are working on. These communications will help guide you into a deeper understanding and more efficient use of all the energies that are available to you.

The following story, although it includes the use of elements, illustrates many other Alchemical Healing techniques as well. I have been teaching in Hamburg for many years, sponsored by an associate, Hiltrud (Anugama) Marg, one of the elder Reiki masters of Germany and an Alchemical Healing instructor. Many of the same community of people have returned year after year. Among this circle is a particularly heroic young woman, R., who has been battling cancer throughout the time I have been traveling there, and in all the years she has only missed one class.

There have been several years when I was sure that I was seeing and working with R. for the last time, for she was so frail I did not know how she could survive. Also, it was a four-story climb to the place where we held our classes.

In 1997 I offered a first-level Alchemical Healing class. Leaning heavily on another student and on her crutches, R. could barely make it up the stairs. She would arrive at the top breathless and would have to be helped inside. She needed assistance both sitting and rising. On the second day I decided to start with a demonstration and to use

R. to show the class the techniques of the first level. She was suffering terribly, mostly from the pituitary cancer that had long since spread to other parts of her body. I was disturbed when I saw how she had deteriorated since the last time I had been in Hamburg. She is as sweet as an angel and carries her suffering with grace and dignity.

We started with her hips, which had been troubling her for several years. I set her in Earth and warmed things up, then burned away the corrosion with Fire and some Air for more heat. Because I was teaching first level, I did not use Akasha. Instead I rinsed with Water and set up drains at the soles of her feet. I set the healing in Earth after she could feel the movement of the bones, and that part was done.

Next I worked on the tailbone. I used elements and then invited Bear in to help. I can't remember the combination of what we did to ease the pain, but the vertebrae slipped back into place, and the pain disappeared.

R.'s heart, weakened by chemotherapy, had problems circulating the blood. Her lungs were filling with liquid. At her heart I used the wood violet and another herb that came to me when I asked for help (be open to guidance as well as inspiration). I later learned that the wood violet is a good ally in working with cancers of all types, although it is most known for assisting with skin cancer. R. expressed immediate relief from the infusion of the herbal spirits.

Next we began working on the brain, and I was called to use the herbs gota kola and pau d'arco. The pau d'arco came in on a smell and I told her to pay close attention for the message from this wisdom.

I used my Fire finger to penetrate the skull and brain mass to get to the pituitary gland where the tumor was located. R. is so sensitive that she was able to inform me of the progress; she could feel every subtle move of my hand, even though I never touched her. When the energy reached the tumor it transformed into a laser. Everyone in the room was momentarily paralyzed, unable to move because the focus had to be held so intensely. As I continued to point toward the tumor, I suddenly was aware of a tiny light, with a tinge of red in it, at the precise point where I was directing the energy.

R. was able to signal when she felt that the tumor was gone. I used Water to rinse and filled the void with healing herbs. It took some time before R. was able to return to ordinary consciousness enough to speak. She rested on the floor with pillows for quite some time. The whole process—a culmination of years of work on her part with the help of the many other healers—took less than two hours. When I offered her my hand, she rose easily to a standing position. Then I put on "Renewal" from my *Tribal Alchemy* CD and we danced, all of us, for the entire piece, about twenty-five minutes. It was a remarkable moment—there was R., dancing, the entire time. This was a miracle that left no doubt. For the rest of the afternoon she sat up comfortably, and when she left she was walking alone down the stairs, carrying her crutches.

A note of follow-up: It has been six years since the session above. R. is still alive and fighting, although there have been some close brushes with death along the way. My hat is off to this brave warrior!

11
HEALING WITH
SPIRIT ALLIES

THERE IS A CENTRAL PLACE where all the spokes of the wheel of life, all of the paths, come together. The deeper and more fully you experience a single path, the more directly you are able to come to the center where all roads converge. The way of each culture and each tradition has its own color and texture. Its unique imagery adds beauty and interest to the mandala of the creation.

Huna was, for me, a path that I could follow toward the center where all the paths of my personal journey intersected and lent strength to one another. Correspondences between various cultural and traditional views began to emerge, and I was energized by the similarities between Polynesian, Egyptian, and Native American traditions.

My strongest guidance comes from spirit allies with whom I have built relationships over time. They appear in many forms—as deities, animal totems, plant spirits, crystals, and archetypes. These are intelligent spirits that express the attributes and qualities of our natural world, in forms imbued with cultural symbolism, myth, and tradition. Because of the folklore and traditional beliefs associated with these entities, there is a remarkable consistency in all people's experience of them, regardless of their degree of study or practice.

At the base of alchemy is the relationship of elements, and all spirit allies have elemental associations. For example, all winged creatures are associated with the element Air, whether they are eagles or fairies, winged goddesses or members of the angelic host. Air speaks of wisdom and truth, mental facility, communication, beauty. When the winged allies enter they often bring messages. For example, it was the Archangel Gabriel that brought the Koran in its entirety to Mohammed. Some totems are obviously a blend of elements. Hippopotamus is a good example, because it is a massive creature of earth, living at the intersection of earth and water. Reptiles are often a blend of elements, as are sea mammals. Alchemy speaks of the transformative result that occurs in the mixing of the elements. Now that you have a grasp of the meaning of the elements and can begin to perceive the spirit allies elementally, you can see what situations they might best respond to.

When we practice Alchemical Healing we can invoke various things such as the pure elements, the energies of various deities, nature spirits, plants, animals, rocks and minerals, and even the spirits of colors; all of these things are tools in our medicine bag. When we work with these allies, we come to realize that they are not just fanciful ideas, but are the organized consciousness embodied in each of life's forms, more or less concretized in accordance with the realms in which they reside.

ANIMAL TOTEMS

Animal totems are reliable members of any healing team. A novice can discover their totemic qualities both through reading the many books on the subject, and through direct experience using shamanic journey work. I recommend developing relationships with the ones you encounter in these pages as well as with any other animal totems that you may come across as the work progresses.

Totems embody the unique and accumulated experience and innate attributes of particular animal species on an archetypal scale.

Their consciousness becomes available to us when we merge with the collective intelligence of our Higher Selves, according to our intentions and the needs of the moment. For example, throughout our evolution, we have had relationships with Bear. That ongoing relationship has imprinted our memory at a cellular level. The attributes associated with Bear are therefore universal. When we invoke Bear, we bring to awareness the awesome power of the intelligence and evolutionary process that created this powerful species, as well as our cellular memory of ancient relationships, regardless of where on the planet we are from. This energy is already organized for us and when we bring it into the healing process, we are bringing a vast intelligence into the energetic form with which we are working. This is true of all archetypes.

From Hopi *kachinas* in Arizona to the Puma in Peru, the Cobra and Vulture in Egypt, and the Elephant in India, animals are revered and acknowledged as intelligent beings. Across cultures and continents, the same totemic species take on similar roles. The prankster energies of Trickster, who teaches by making a fool of any- and everyone, are expressed in many Native American traditions by Coyote, and in Japan by Fox. The energies of Cobra in Egypt and Rattlesnake in North America function in similar ways. Both are Great Awakeners! And on most continents, except where Christianity has vilified them, snakes are seen as a universal symbol of healing and energy, and of immortality and protection.

Everywhere we look in nature we find our own attributes—and those we wish to emulate—mirrored back to us in other life forms. Since prehistoric times, clans have often identified themselves with the animal totems they revere.

Our introduction to power animals may come in many ways. We can dream of them, encounter them in our lives in the wild or through recurrent appearances and synchronicity, or they can spontaneously, sometimes repetitively, arise in our meditations, inner journeys and quests. Totems can be introduced through a journey process such as the visualization that follows, or a shamanic drum journey. Journeying with a power animal creates a resonance between the consciousness of the totem and our human consciousness. This inner resonance allows us to bring into the work the intelligence, qualities, aspects, and worldview of the totem. While it is possible to work with these allies without prior initiation, building relationships does help us access their full power. Initiation into the animal's power often comes directly from the ally, either during the initial encounter or at some point during the development of a relationship. Totemic initiations are powerful interactions that install the energetic configuration of the totem into your own energetic system at a deeper level.

Sometimes your experience of a totem will take the form of transfiguration, during which you experience the shape as well as the viewpoint and attributes of the totem in yourself. Merging with a totem offers a profound opportunity to experience and utilize the power of your ally. For example, merging with Eagle will allow you to fly, and in so doing have a different perspective, a loftier view of whatever situation you are working on. Becoming a lioness will give you the benefit of her discriminatory faculties and acute sense of sight.

Whatever totemic or spirit energies you employ, it is important to keep these relationships vital with your attention. Visit and work with them often. It may help to have pictures of them, statuary, stuffed animals, or something in your home to remind you of their presence in your life in a physical way.

Although every person has a power animal with whom he or she has a special affinity, you can also develop relationships with many animal totems. Often there is a subconscious link between you and your power animal that expresses itself in your love for its species, even though you are not always aware of its influence in your life. When you develop a conscious relationship with a totem, it becomes your ally. Totems are powerful messengers, healers, and protectors, and they bring great benefit to those who build and maintain such relationships. Some of the most prominent allies used in Alchemical Healing are described in depth in *Power Animal Meditations*. The following journey will take you to meet whatever power animal is relevant for you to work with at the moment.

It is important to remember that many of the animals that we encounter and work with are fierce and wild in nature. As we enter into relationships with them, regardless of whether they are fierce or timid creatures, we must approach them with respect and honor the qualities that they share with us. Notice the initial emotions that your totem evokes in you, and strive for recognition of the joy and comfort this relationship can bring. The totem you will meet can be of any species, and is here to show you something about your life, and perhaps your healing work.

Your experience with your totem will be enhanced if you are willing to give back. Attention and gratitude are always welcome, and you will find that innovative offerings will be well received. Be willing to return to further develop the bond that is created during this initial introduction.

JOURNEY

ANIMAL TOTEM JOURNEY

Smudge and create an appropriate, comfortable space. Close your eyes, ground and center, using the breath to fill your belly on the inhale, and then exhale downward through your tailbone to connect yourself with the earth. . . .

Devote attention to your heart flame, directing love to make it grow and to spread its radiance throughout your being, filling you with warmth and light. . . .

Stir the waters within your golden cauldron. . . . Notice as the waters rise to meet the flame in your heart, and experience the conversion as the water meets the fire and turns to steam. . . .

The steam rises, opening the shamanic passageway at your throat to fill your head. Place your entire attention within the steam.

As it gathers in your head, it will lift your consciousness up through your crown and into your light body. . . .

It is dark. The first sense that awakens is smell. . . . Then you notice the temperature. . . . You are starting to get an idea of where on the planet you are. . . . There are sounds. . . . The senses you have awakened intensify. Tune in and concentrate on them. . . . You realize your eyes have been closed. Open your inner eyes and look around. . . . There is a sound; something is nearing. Listen. What is it? It pauses. . . . You are getting more and more information about your surroundings, even the time of the day or night. . . . There is that sound again. Your totem animal approaches you. . . . When you turn your head toward it, you find yourself looking directly into the eyes of your totem. . . .

This power animal is here to help you, to show you something about your life. . . . Open your heart in greeting as you request an experience. . . .

Follow your totem. Watch. . . . Listen. . . . Feel to the fullest. . . . Learn from what is offered. . . . *[Long pause . . .]*

It is time to return. . . . Take a moment to consider what you can give back to this totem, and be sure to offer your gratitude for the experience and the lessons learned. . . .

When you feel complete for now, your totem (or Thoth) will assist you back through your crown and into your physical body.

Ground and center. . . .

Your totem will always be available to guide and help you.*

ARCHETYPES AND DEITIES

Deities are culturally created representations of fundamental principles that are unchangeable, incorruptible, and real. We relate to deities to understand those principles in ourselves. In so doing, we

---

*A version of this journey is recorded in my CD *Tribal Alchemy*.

honor even those aspects of our nature that frighten us or show us our shadow side.

Deities dwell in each person's consciousness as the personal and cultural symbols of the archetypes, which are expressions of basic and fundamental ideas. For example, the Great Mother is a concept that, when personified, becomes Isis, Mary, or Tara. The Greek Goddess Hecate is a cultural interpretation of an archetypal Crone.

In most world cultures divine beings originate in the realm of nature. Egypt's gods and goddesses maintain obvious alignments with the natural world; for example Hathor appears as a cow, or a sycamore tree, as a turquoise gemstone, or as the sky itself. Other cultures likewise acknowledge similar ties between divine beings and the natural world: Ganesha, the elephant god of the Hindus; Oshun, water goddess of the Yoruba tradition; and White Buffalo Woman of the Native American tradition. In this way the symbols express the deeper meanings and powers in each belief system. In such worship no intercessor is placed between oneself and the divine nature manifest in the world. The individual can attain direct communication and communion with the Divine.

By exploring these and other systems, one begins to see the similarities at the core of these varying theologies. In Egypt the cow who ploughs the earth and offers her milk and meat for sustenance is also the cow goddess, Hathor, from whose breasts flow the nourishment of the Milky Way, the *mana* from the celestial river of life. In the tradition of the Native American Plains tribes the totemic Buffalo gives the people sustenance in the forms of food, shelter, tools, and clothing, while the divine White Buffalo Woman gives nourishment to the spirit of the people with her gifts of the sacred Pipe and ceremonies. Hathor and White Buffalo Woman are more like cousins than sisters, but they are essentially related.

Other deities play important roles in our work. Thoth oversees and orchestrates Alchemical Healing. Kuan Yin, the Oriental goddess of compassion and mercy, and Sekhmet, the quintessentially compassionate Egyptian goddess of healing, are indispensable resources, both for healing support and for specific techniques. When I invoke my guides and helpers I invite any who wish to participate to come forward, and I always honor the deities that have offered their assistance. My relationships with these divinities have been built over time, again based on attention and reverence. As I did, you may find yourself with a natural affinity toward one or another, and it will be up to you to determine when and whether to call upon a particular deity.

My life experience has introduced me to a large variety of belief systems, yet the ones that have most attracted me are those of Native Americans and ancient Egyptians. Although superficially they seem worlds apart, I am continually amazed by the similarities.

Before colonization there were about five hundred separate languages across the diverse climates and conditions that make up North America. Yet there were certain consistencies among most all tribes. Each tribe lived close to the elements and had a deep understanding and respect for all aspects of nature. In order to survive, they had to understand the ways of the animals and plants and live in harmony with their surroundings. Each tribe had a rich mythology and inherent wisdom passed through storytelling from generation to generation.

The most obvious similarity between the high civilization of Egypt and the so-called primitive indigenous cultures of America is the totemic quality of the gods. Both cultures deified nature and imagined their gods in the forms of animals. But the similarities do not end there.

We commonly think of Native America as shamanistic. Ancient Egypt was also shamanistic at its core. Her most widely quoted myth, the story of Isis and Osiris, conveys the classic shamanic journey of life, death, and dismemberment. Re-membering and resurrection of life occur through the magic and power of love. This fundamental precept was acted out in physical form in the early dynastic period, when the bones of the dead were actually separated and scrubbed before being returned to their original skeletal shape as part of their funerary rites.

In places like Peru, where there are vast remains of Incan cities and temples, icons were cast in gold rather than carved on stone walls. Only that which escaped the crucibles of the conquistadors remains to tell us of their reverence for nature, the animals, and plants.

Throughout Egypt, exquisite bas-relief carvings cover almost every available surface of the temples, depicting their gods in the stories that have held the history and deepest meanings of their cosmology for thousands of years. The Cairo Museum contains a rich selection of statuary that depicts many of the people and gods of Egypt. Many of these were carved by artisan-priests trained in the magical traditions of working with stone to imbue it with spiritual essence, or *ka*.

The word for a deity in Egypt is *neter*, or the family of *neteru;* these are derivatives of nature, or *nether*. The Coptic Egyptians use the word *netcher* for nature. The neteru represent the principles of life that make up who we are and how we behave. To know the divinities is to know ourselves. Then, when we need to express a certain principle in our lives in specific situations, we can draw upon the living energy of that principle that has been nurtured and made accessible by our attention.

A statue of the goddess Sekhmet stands in a small chapel at the temple of Karnak in Egypt. When in the presence of this statue, one gets a sense of the original intention placed in the stone. It still emanates the energy attributed to the archetype that Sekhmet represents. This lioness goddess of Egypt who exemplifies the feminine fire of destruction and creation is also the deeply compassionate healer. She is one of the most deeply felt and strongest allies in Alchemical Healing. She has the fierceness, intelligence, strength, power, and discrimination of the lioness. Her keen senses can be applied to whatever challenge is at hand. When I am engaged in difficult or dangerous healing work, I might call on Sekhmet and invite her into my body to help me. She also gives me courage when I am feeling frightened or timid, and adds her fire to my own to increase the power of my actions. When I call on Sekhmet, I am calling on those aspects of *myself* that are intrinsic, although often easier to perceive if they have been objectified in this manner.

Recently I worked with a woman who wanted to meet the Egyptian goddess Sekhmet, because Sekhmet had appeared to her years earlier at a time when this person felt uncomfortable responding. This time, when we journeyed for direction, she described a doglike personage with a black face, pointy nose and ears, and piercing yellow eyes. I immediately recognized this ally as Anubis, the jackal god of Egypt, opener of the way and guardian of the underworld. I introduced him, describing his attributes—his ability to protect equally in the dark and the light, his keen sensitivities and loyalty, his functions as Lord of Embalming, protector of miscarried and abandoned children, and guardian of the treasuries in the tombs. I also said that I found him helpful in communicating with those who have crossed over.

It is important to note that I did not call Anubis. He appeared because, as it turned out, he knew what this woman really needed, and when I suggested that she follow him to find out what he had come to show her, he led her on a wonderful journey of self-discovery. Afterward she felt more at ease and confident regarding the challenges that originally brought her to call me.

This is part of the mystery and magic of this work. We become witnesses to the alchemical healing process of others. With practice we learn to follow the clues we are given and help our clients to perceive the choices available to them. By our experience, we guide them into empowering relationships that will sustain them long after we leave. Once the connection is made, our task is to get out of the way and let this new relationship develop. We can encourage this developing relationship by providing valuable exercises or homework that encourages the work to continue. These new internal relationships will grow stronger with attention.

I stress the importance of communicating with and getting to know the various deities and archetypes because it is important that you forge relationships with whoever can help you in the healing work. Each consciousness has a particular unique resonance. When you align your awareness with the resonance of any being, you create a connection to that entity that is yours alone. The combination of your resonance with the archetype creates a unique configuration. For example, if you tune into the archetype of the wise old Crone and you see a wrinkled, withered grandma with long white braids, then that is your energetic key to the Crone. If someone else sees a wizened old woman who fades into a vulture and back into a woman, that person's visualization is equally valid. You will only learn to identify the key by working with the archetype and getting to know the form it presents to you. As you explore the possibilities of these connections through the work of Alchemical Healing, you often encounter unique beings who, with a little research, you will discover to be part of an ancient tradition reaching through time to connect with you.

My husband has a very close relationship with Thoth, developed over years of working with me and helping me to bring in these teachings. When we communicate with Thoth, he appears in many guises. Sometimes he even shapeshifts into other forms altogether. Over time and through experience, Mark's relationship with him has been refined and personalized so that regardless of the form Thoth takes, he can be distinguished from any other entity that might assume his place. Mark can make these distinctions because he listens and pays attention to his inner sense of Thoth's presence. When he "goes in" with the intention of seeing Thoth, he sometimes is presented with someone else. He knows, by what he calls "the flavor," that this is not just another aspect of Thoth. When this happens, it is up to him to discover the purpose and meaning of this volunteer. When an archetype comes to you in an unusual guise, that guise provides a very important clue to what is needed in that moment, regardless of the form taken.

We all know how to do this practice: consciousness knows how to recognize an essence. But that recognition requires first that a relationship exists; that only happens when your consciousness understands itself to be *at-one* with the archetypal energy. One's ability to relate to the archetype as part of Self is proportional to the intimacy developed in the relationship.

In Mark's case, this intimacy is something that he brought into this life and learned to see. We are all part of what one could call Thoth's *family*, and yet Thoth is an aspect of each of us—our Higher Self, and our wiser Self—and from Thoth's perspective there is a shared energetic resonance and a shared sense of intention and purpose. Those of us drawn to this work form an active collective on earth at this time. Through continued interaction we can learn more about from whence we came and what we came here to accomplish.

The student who wishes to understand these archetypes as principles of creation will open lines of communication with them. This open line helps bring forth the energies of the archetypes, deities, and totem allies when you practice healing. The more you practice, and the more attention you give to them, the more immediately they show up. They can also then serve as guides throughout your spiritual development.

THE HEALING TEAM

When you think you are alone, it becomes a huge responsibility and a lonely and daunting task to attempt to heal others, or even yourself. Understand this: The healing is not accomplished by or because of you alone. When you know that you are part of something larger, with other perspectives to take into account, then healing feels like a joyful dance with a diverse array of partners keeping it endlessly interesting. Whether you perceive your spirit guides and totems as inside you or separate from you, when you honor and allow their intelligence to enhance your healing work, new opportunities and possibilities present themselves. You are no longer limited by your own skill; you can take advantage of the natural abilities and talents of other life forms. From the lowly maggot, who is known to have been an ally to wounded soldiers in battle, entering and cleaning their infected wounds, to the lofty flying eagle that gives us discriminating perspective from high above, each form has unique attributes that you can apply to many healings. With your intention, attention, and discrimination, you can easily find the ally that is the best choice for the work at hand. Often you have an idea of what needs to be done. If a person has a broken bone in a place that cannot be splinted, such as a collarbone, you might look for an ally who can build a structure to protect it while the bone has time to knit. Comfrey, or "knit bone," is an obvious plant ally you could use ethereally and also physically, in tea, tinctures, or capsules, to support the etheric work. You could use the element Earth, which helps to build structure. You could get creative and imaginative, too, by looking for a living being whose attributes could be useful. Coral comes to mind, especially for a slow-healing break. You could ask the coral to build itself around the injured area to hold it secure. Another possibility would be Spider, who could weave a supportive web around the bone, or Snake, who could wrap itself around the area to hold it in place while it is mending.

Conversely, deities and totems sometimes come unbidden. There are times when you might not feel comfortable talking with the person you are working on about what you are seeing, yet you may be having a regular movie running in your head. The visual experiences can be as vague as a shadowing suggestion, or as vivid as a Technicolor three-dimensional video, complete with smells and soundtrack.

Kathryn Ravenwood, a wonderful massage therapist and healer who is teaching Alchemical Healing in Washington state, had this experience:

> One of my clients, N., came in while she was having a miscarriage. She was bleeding and in a lot of pain. Because she is a Latino Catholic, I was nervous about offending her with the more esoteric aspects of Alchemical Healing. I decided I would only send in energy to help stop the bleeding. As soon as I put my hands on her, however, I discovered I could see quite vividly into another dimension. We were at a beautiful lagoon or pool in Africa where hippos live. N. was in the water and as I

observed the scene two hippos came up to her and cradled her there in the water between their huge bodies, supporting her. Their energy was blissful and loving. They kept holding her and empathizing with her over the loss of her child. They obviously were sad with and for her. I did not feel comfortable with telling N. what I was seeing.

The hippos, one on each side of N., started squeezing her a little, undulating back and forth, squishing her between the two of them while she continued floating between them in the pool. Blood started pouring out of her. All the dried blood and mucous and gunk from the miscarriage that had not come out of her body slipped out now into the pool. The hippos kept lovingly and gently squishing her while they swayed back and forth, pushing her between them. They were right with her, the force of their bodies gently squeezing the remaining gore out of her until the entire pool was red with blood.

When the miscarriage was over and she was all cleaned out, the blood flowed away and the water became clear again. When N. had bathed and rinsed in the clear water, I thanked the hippos and returned my consciousness to the room where we began the healing session.

Kathryn could not bring herself to tell N. what she had witnessed, and when she asked N. her experience, she simply thanked her, said she felt better, and left. The next week, N. returned and demanded to know what Kathryn had done to her. When Kathryn shared the story of her vision, N. was quite moved that the hippos had helped her in that way, even if she herself did not see them. The bleeding had stopped right away, and all pain had vanished.

It should be noted that there is an Egyptian goddess, Taueret, who is a composite of the hippo, lioness, crocodile, and human with pendulous breasts. This goddess is a midwife, and is present at all physical births. Talismans of her image were carried by those who wanted to be pregnant, for fertility, and by those who were already pregnant, for protection. She appears in *Power Animal Meditations* as the hippopotamus, where she offers a wonderful Journey of Rebirth.

I too had an experience of a hippo coming as Taueret during a miscarriage that I was attending many years ago. It was one of the true miracles that I've witnessed, for with the assistance of this warm and loving hippo (do not try this in the wild), the miscarriage itself was aborted, and the resulting child is now a healthy and vibrant teenager.

BEAR ON THE TEAM!

Bear has appeared many times to come to my aid during healings. Sometimes I invoke her, and sometimes she simply shows up. Regardless, she always provides creative solutions that I would not have thought of on my own.

Bear, a fierce protector of her own cubs, loves children, and can be called upon most any time you are working with children. She can be counted upon to be playful and caring, and instill in children a sense of trust and safety.

Bear also knows herbal medicine. If you think an herbal medicine is needed but don't know which one, you can always go to Crone or Bear for a remedy. These remedies might come in a variety of forms—salve, balm, poultice, tincture, or tea. Always remember to thank the spirit of the herb that is given, and offer back a blast of life force energy blended with a large dose of love for the plant and its family.

One time while demonstrating techniques for a class, I worked with a student who suffered from severe diabetes. Lynn had been blind for twelve years, the result of the experimental laser surgery of the time. He could only distinguish light and shadow. The doctors had removed his lenses as well, so he had no peripheral vision, nor could he gain that part of his sight back. He did have the conviction that he could heal and was eager for the opportunity to try using the methods we were learning. Once the energetic connection was established between us, I took him on a guided visualization to see who might come forward to help. Two large brown she-bears came clearly into view in Lynn's inner landscape and were also visible to the other students. One bear sharpened her claw on a stone. Lynn described for us very clearly, and we all watched, while this bear very carefully approached his eyes, then used her sharpened claw to lift the scar tissue off his retina. Bears cannot retract their claws, so they are very deft. It was amazing to witness. Each of us could feel it, and Lynn was able to articulate his experience of the touch of the bear's claw on his most sensitive eyes. I should note here that there was no fear, for he felt an immediate and natural trust in these spirit bears.

When the first bear completed her part, she stepped back, and the other bear came forward and handed Lynn a vial of liquid to drink. He was able to taste the herbs that made up this medicine, even though the drink was etheric. Intuition indicated that we wait for a few minutes for the potion to take effect. When we refocused, Lynn had traveled back in time to the Middle Ages to an event that seemed to be the original experience that caused a pattern of blindness to recur lifetime after lifetime. He found himself in the midst of a horribly barbaric war, and he recalled how it felt to be in the service of others and to gouge out the eyes of their enemies, including the eyes of children. The vision played like a vivid memory in his mind. He could feel the emotions that upset him so much that, in that other life, he raised a firebrand to his own eyes and blinded himself. He related this experience in great detail and even saw himself being cared for by those he had injured. With the memory of that past life, he was able to release the pattern that had been imprinted on his DNA.

When the vision was over and he had made the changes internally, he thanked the bears and the healing was complete. He slowly opened his eyes and looked around. Even without lenses, he could see the shapes of the flowers and the silhouette of the house. It was remarkable to witness his elation. The following week he visited his doctor to have his sight measured. The result of his efforts was that he had regained 20 percent of his vision and completely cured his glaucoma.

ANOTHER BEAR STORY

We were doing a sweat lodge, and George was having trouble dealing with the heat. He left the lodge after the third round and went to the house. While we were doing the last round, my husband went to check on him. He found George on the floor, retching. He helped him to lie down and became alarmed when George went into convulsions. When we came in after the sweat, Mark was ministering to him as best he could. My initial reaction to the scene was fear, followed by a strong urge to get him to the hospital as fast as possible.

I paused long enough to take a deep breath and ask for help. I was immediately aware of the presence of an old grandmother bear. I was also reminded that I was involved in a sacred activity, and that the cure would most likely come from a source similar to the cause. I knew that in this situation I had to maintain faith in the magic. So I decided to try the alchemical work first, with a hard eye on reality, so that if things persisted or worsened I could get him to the hospital right away.

Because he had not lost consciousness, I was able to introduce George to Bear quite easily, and he was able to articulate to us his experience as it was happening. As soon as he saw the bear, George knew he would be okay. She gathered him into her loving embrace and offered him a cup of some kind of medicinal herbal tea. He drank the tea, and within five minutes he was back to normal and ready to head for home! We kept him at our house for a while, anyway, just to make sure he was clearheaded and well grounded before he drove home.

SPIDER MEDICINE

I had been working with totems and Alchemical Healing for many years before Spider joined the team as a powerful healing ally. When she made her rather dramatic entrance during a ceremony I was doing with my husband, I knew by the flavor of the experience I was in for a good ride. I had always honored Grandmother Spider as the weaver of creation, and she often showed up during my planetary healing classes. I had an opportunity to work with her during an

Alchemical Healing class I was teaching at Bo Clark's center, Hawks Above, in Cloudland, Georgia.

For the demonstration of techniques I enlisted Kim, a young woman who had been in a serious horse accident. Her knee was still discolored, swollen, and giving her severe chronic pain. I connected to her in the way I usually do, although from the start my intention was to invoke Spider. I drew Akasha around her and she was able to see herself as a tree, an image that she told me later was common to her experience. I used all the appropriate techniques to remove the original trauma and the lingering swelling (as presented in the chapter on healing techniques) before we entered into the journey part of the healing.

Although I invoked Spider, it was leaf cutter ants that showed up to begin the tedious task of removing, piece by piece, the edema that had collected there. They carried the black sludge deep into the earth. When the ants had completed their task, I flushed out the knee with water. Spider appeared, and very delicately wove a web of silk thread to encase the revamped knee, providing a structural bandage to protect the knee as it healed. The spider's web, stronger than steel, wrapped around the tendons and joint capsule like a cocoon, supporting them firmly yet gently.

The scar, readily apparent earlier in Kim's vision, was entirely gone; in its place now was Spider, in the center of the web bandage.

Following this demonstration the pain was gone for some time, and the swelling and purple bruising reduced tremendously. Kim's mobility greatly increased and the knee has not been stiff since. Spider has proven to be an important, ongoing ally on Kim's spiritual path.

PLANT SPIRITS

Plants are our most potent allies for healing. Most all of the medicines in the modern medical pharmacopoeia are derivatives of or synthesized from plants. For example, aspirin comes from the willow tree. Digitalis, a heart medicine, is derived from the beautiful foxglove flower. Taxol, used in chemotherapy for breast cancer, is extracted from the bark of the yew tree. The list could go on, and would seem endless were it not for the fact that our potential medicinal resources are dwindling, along with our rainforests and other natural environments that are being urbanized or overdeveloped for grazing lands, agriculture, or managed forests. Many plants known for their curative powers, such as American ginseng, are gathered for profit alone, and are being exploited for their cash value to the point of extinction.

Healing herbs are a basic element of Alchemical Healing; yet we do not require the physical plant in order to work with its magic. More than any other aspect of this healing form, the work with the plant spirits conveys the power of subtle energies.

EXERCISE

Healing with Plant Spirits

Almost every healing can be enhanced with herbal energy. For those who have some herbal knowledge, it is a simple matter to call in the power of the plants with which you are familiar. If you know the name of a plant that is helpful for a condition that you are working with, you can call it by name. Picture the plant in your mind as you reach out with your hand, palm up, to receive its energy, knowing that the *in potentia* reality is only a thought away. As you hold out your hand, mentally greet the spirit of the plant and offer a blast of life force energy to its species, its family, with a prayer for its health and continuance. Then ask the spirit to come to you and provide the attributes that would be useful for the healing in progress. When you feel the weight of the spirit medicine in your hand, direct it into the place in the body where you are working, or to a place that provides a conduit to where the plant medicine needs to be.

For example, comfrey is a strong healing plant with which I have a solid relationship. Its folk name is *knit bone* because it contains an active ingredient called allantoin, a substance that helps to bind cells together. Comfrey is a very versatile plant, and as its name suggests, it brings comfort wherever it is directed. It helps heal burns, lungs, cuts, and abrasions, and has antibiotic properties. If I were using the physical plant I might mash the leaves to make a poultice, make an infusion of the leaves for tea, or gather the mucilaginous goo from the roots to apply directly to burns, lacerations, or infections. I might also dry the root to powder for capsules.

Although any herbal first-aid kit that I would own would contain comfrey, most of the time I am relying on my healing hands and my mind, and so I consider comfrey as one of my most valued friends. I often ask the spirit of the plant for its powers to heal wounds and burns, to bring comfort to bruises and traumatized places, and to mend bones. I am quite specific when communicating with the spirit. "Hello old friend, Comfrey. Will you please bring your healing powers to this work. My friend here is in need of your abilities to mend her bone quickly, for she is in pain." I wait until I feel the weight of the plant spirit in my hand; I then direct it with my hand and actually make the motions of wrapping it around the broken bone. The effect, especially with such injuries as fractured bones, is usually felt immediately, even through a cast. I recommend waiting until the bone has been set properly to do this work, because you don't want the bones to bind together before they are joined where they belong.

I have a limited amount of herbal knowledge; yet there are a number of plant spirit allies with whom I have made powerful relationships. When I am aware that the condition requires help from plants that I do not know, I go to Bear or Crone, the wise old woman archetype who knows the ways of the herbs, and ask for help. Or I can ask, simply, "whoever wishes to step forward to help me with this healing, please come forward and give me the herb that I need." As you practice, you will find that the archetypes and spirit helpers are right there for you as soon as you set your intention to do the healing work. If you are not educated regarding the names and properties of medicinal herbs, you must rely upon your ability to perceive at the more intuitive levels. Because I do not see or hear clairvoyantly, I have learned to trust Bear and Crone. The results have been consistent and profound.

In illustration of this trust, I am reminded of a time some years ago when I picked up a friend at the airport to go to a healing gathering. As we drove toward the mountains, she complained of stomach cramps, which she attributed to the meager diet of airplane food. I reached over to generate energy into her stomach, but it didn't seem to have any effect. I knew there was a plant medicine that would heal her quickly, but I didn't know what it was. So I called on Crone, and asked for a remedy. I was aware of her presence, although I could not see her directly, and knew that she was preparing something. Within a moment I felt her put something my hand, and when I turned my hand to place it over my friend's stomach and direct the medicine into her, the effect was immediate: the pain stopped and the cramping relaxed.

The healing possibilities of working with plant allies are endless. For example, genital herpes is a very common and miserable problem, for which there is really no consistent cure. It returns periodically to plague its host, and in between bouts usually lives in the person's spinal column. I have had considerable experience working with both genital herpes and the related blisters that develop around the mouth (cold sores). For both I use the same thing: cayenne. To physically use cayenne requires great care, because it can feel as though it is burning the soft tissue in both mouth and genitals. It can be done, carefully, if you keep to the actual blister. But a much easier and equally effective option is to ask for help from the spirit of the cayenne plant, then place its energy where the blisters are occurring. This is especially powerful when done at the very beginning of a herpes outbreak; however, even if the sores have opened it can speed the healing considerably. (Never touch a person's herpes blister directly, as it spreads by contact.)

HEALING WITH TREES

We humans have a wonderful symbiotic relationship with trees, especially obvious in the oxygen/carbon dioxide exchange. One of the best ways to open communication with a tree is to share breath

consciously. We can accomplish this both on the inner planes as well
as in the physical world.

EXERCISE

Becoming a Tree

Take a moment to ground and center yourself, and feed your
heart flame. . . . In the expanding light of your heart flame, you
will find yourself in a meadow, a grove of trees, or forest, or simply standing before a familiar tree.

Approach your tree and allow yourself to acknowledge the
connection that develops as a result of your intention and attention. Greet this tree from your heart. As you feel yourself come
into resonance with the tree, notice how the sharing of breath,
which is a natural function of our relationship with trees regardless of our awareness, can be a rich, nourishing experience. . . .

When resonance is established, it is easy to step into the tree
and feel yourself within its sturdy trunk, aware of its roots deep
within the earth, drawing energy from the soil and water. You
can actually feel yourself as the tree, aspects of your own body
superimposed within the tree's body, the tree reflecting your
health quite specifically in its leaves, its bark, and the way it holds
itself. . . . From within the tree you will begin to understand why
you have chosen this particular species of tree, with its individual
characteristics. Just as the history of the tree is evident in the
direction and growth of its trunk and branches, so your own history is delineated in this tree form you have adopted now.

The longer you remain in this relationship, the more details
will emerge. . . . When it is time, step out of the tree and ground
and center yourself back in your physical body.

This practice is useful for therapists and healers, who can learn to very quickly superimpose their clients onto their individual tree bodies as a method of gathering information. You can learn a great deal about your client's health from the health of his or her tree, from its deciduous or evergreen nature, from its season, the vibrancy of its color, and from the texture and quality of the leaves and of any fruit that appears. Even the wildlife that may surround the tree can bring messages and clues about the health of the person.

Trees are willing servants to the healing work. Sometimes when I am working with particularly virulent energies, I will use water as a medium to hold the energies I've removed (see Chapter 16) and carry it out to a tree. After asking permission of the tree—I have never had one refuse—I will offer the water at the base of the tree with a prayer for the transformation of the undesirable spirit into its highest potential.

When you are distraught or holding trauma, a fast, effective way to safely conduct the excess emotion out of yourself is to approach a tree in the physical world, share breath with it consciously for a moment, and ask the tree if it will help you deal with the emotions you are feeling. Place both hands on the tree trunk, or the outer leaves if you can't get close to the trunk. You can hug your tree if that feels more comfortable. The tree will draw out your excess emotion, whether it is grief, pain, or anger. This can be a very cathartic experience that stimulates you to cry or even wail, or it can happen swiftly and with great ease.

My first experience of this happened spontaneously many years ago, before I had any understanding of the process. I was extremely distraught about some family matters and went to a redwood grove to seek solace. There was an ancient tree that had been hollowed at the base, probably from a lightning strike. I entered this womblike tree cave and immediately felt safe and secure. It was as if the walls of the tree formed a huge magnet, which pulled the misery right out of me in a flood of tears that, although it did not solve the problem, left me cleansed of my overwrought emotions and much more able to deal with my situation.

Years later a Kahuna friend, Henry, shared a similar technique with me that was most effective and validated my own previous discovery. We were working together in a situation where we were not able to be outside, so we had to connect with the chosen tree from a distance to accomplish the same thing, and it was equally effective. That time we were working on René, a man who had been caught in an explosion in San Francisco in which nine people died. It was ten weeks later, and René was so traumatized from the accident that he could barely walk, although all obvious exterior symptoms had disappeared directly. We were in an apartment complex where the only tree was outside, within view from the window but not directly accessible for our purposes. We had him connect psychically with the tree, and it helped significantly to pull out the fear and emotion that was still locked within his body. Henry and I then worked on his auric field to smooth and make peace with the chaotic energies that still swirled around him, following which we all retired for the night. The next morning René awoke and put his clothes on before he even realized what he was doing. He had not been able to put his pants on without assistance since before the explosion.

Recently I was working with a professor of psychology who, at sixty-two, is actually very fit. She had suffered a tennis injury to her wrist that, after many months, had not healed. Her orthopedist had determined that it was probably a torn ligament. She also complained of pain and tenderness on the outside of her joints, a problem that her physician was unable to conclusively diagnose.

Guiding her into a light trance, I introduced her to a spontaneous version of a tree meditation. She found herself, then, in the body of a fir tree. As we began observing her relation to this tree, and how its own joints reflected hers, I suddenly remembered the value of tree pitch in healing. My friend Rolling Thunder used to carry around a jar of pine tar ointment that his wife, Spotted Fawn, made. It was the most potent healing ointment I'd ever seen. Black and pungent, it worked for everything from burns to lesions.

I got an intuitive flash that the pitch in the fir tree could not only help heal her joints, but it could also heal and hold her ligament in place. Using a kind of psychic surgical technique, I energetically put the ligament in place and called on her tree's pitch to surround and hold the ligament. Throughout the healing, I also worked with the elements, encasing her wrist in Earth to protect it and using Akasha to find and restore the original pattern of health.

After a few moments, I asked her to carefully check the movement of her wrist for the usual symptoms. No pain! She had been wearing a wrist splint so I suggested she continue wearing it for three days to keep her wrist immobilized in order to set the work we had done.

HEALING WITH CRYSTALS

All gems and minerals have natural attributes that can be worked with by one who is conscious of subtle energy fields. There are a number of books available that speak more directly to these attributes, so I will focus on the most common mineral ally, quartz. Quartz crystals are a time-honored tool of shamans and magicians throughout the world. They hold a program of vibration, and their frequencies can be tuned and sustained, which is why they were used to make the first radios. They are still an important part of the computer world.

Quartz comes in many color varieties, such as amethyst, citrine, and smoky. Each has its subtle difference. Although I have worked with many gems and minerals, of all colors, clear quartz is the most versatile and available.

In scientific terms, quartz is a mineral consisting of the elements silicon and oxygen. These are two of the most plentiful elements on the earth's surface, but in the quartz crystal, these elements are arranged in orderly crystalline patterns. When you work with quartz crystals, your focused intention creates patterns on a minute scale and conducts electricity flowing through that pattern. This is the same principle that makes a computer chip work. Silicon is used in computer chips because it is possible to very precisely tune its electrical characteristics.

The latticed pattern of the atoms within the quartz crystal form an extremely regular and stable molecular configuration. If a subtle vibration were to enter that matrix it would be held there unchanged. Other substances might not hold the vibration because of the random nature of their molecular structure. Focused intention can alter the program, and when you direct strong thought into the crystal, it affects the frequency.

Oh Shinnah first taught me about the magical and healing properties of crystals in 1974. My then husband, Rock, overheard Oh Shinnah saying that I needed a healing crystal. He rummaged about in his belongings and brought out a beautiful quartz crystal that he had dug directly out of the mountains of Switzerland some years before. With that crystal I learned about the healing attributes of quartz.

Oh Shinnah told me that these crystals amplified thought, so I experimented and found them useful. The first time I used a crystal like a microphone was to send a message to Rock. I knew I had left the phone unplugged at our apartment in San Rafael, and I knew that it would take him about an hour to get there. Meanwhile, an important call had come in for him, and I had to reach him by phone. I waited until I could imagine him arriving, then settling down to rest as was his habit. I took the crystal and focused as intently as I could, trying to get him to notice that the phone was unplugged. Then I dialed the number. He answered on the third ring because it was ringing when he plugged it in.

Amplification of intention is one of the main uses of quartz crystals in healing. It is possible to direct your thoughts through the crystal by pointing it toward where you wish to send the energy. A clean, clear point is best for amplifying the healing work. Crystals that you reserve for healing purposes should be clear, with a point that is not damaged. All crystals should be kept clean and if you travel with them they should be protected separately in pouches, preferably silk with padding to keep them from getting chipped or broken. When you get a new quartz crystal, it should be deeply purified by soaking in salted water at least overnight. It should be cleansed in clear water after each healing use.

I have had a number of crystals over the years that I have dedicated to healing. As with the other allies we have spoken of in this chapter, relationships are developed through attention and engagement. I found that when I carried one with me, I would know when it wanted to be involved in the healing work I was doing at the time.

I try to teach healing techniques that can be used without requiring extenuating props, although it is important to honor the spirits with whom one has an affinity. I travel a lot, and it became quite cumbersome to carry a large altar with representations of my allies, and the crystals that I used when I was first doing healing work. I finally determined that I wanted to develop a form that needed nothing but hands, and if those were encumbered, mind. We might not always have the luxury of a sanctuary in which to work and an altar from which to draw energy. It is helpful to remember that we can connect to our allies from wherever we are.

Nevertheless, crystals can be useful, especially if you have developed a relationship with one that you reserve for healing. I remember working on a woman who was very congested from a lingering flu. Her hearing was affected; it felt as if her ears were filled with cotton. I tried all the techniques I could think of to open her ear canal, to no avail. Yet I knew that just a little more power would do it. I picked up an eagle feather and a particularly strong clear quartz point, and called on them for assistance as I focused on the clogged Eustachian tube. The first sound she heard was the swoosh of the eagle feather, as the combined efforts of the energy from my intention, my hands, the crystal, and the feather finally broke through.

★ ☽ ★

When I was first practicing Reiki I used to take my healing crystals to concerts, where I liked to use the powerful energies of the audience and music to magnify whatever healing work I was doing. I would use the crystals to focus the Reiki energy and to amplify my prayers. I had a particularly strong experience at a Grateful Dead concert at Red Rocks, a natural amphitheater in the mountains of Colorado. I was holding a beautiful clear point, shaped like a wand. During the drum solo, I held the crystal before me as I went into trance and prayed with all my heart. There was a strange shift in the movement of the energy, as though the music was attracted to the crystal and moved through it and out from it as though it was a transmitter.

A week or so after this concert, I found myself at a metaphysical church where the minister was doing a demonstration of psychometry, the art of reading an object. She passed a tray around so that people from the congregation could put something on it for her to read. I still had the crystal with me, so I placed it on the tray. The minister held it for a moment in her hands, then looked directly at me and said, "You have prayed with this crystal at a cathedral. I will not repeat your prayers here, but I will tell you that they will be answered."

Bear is an ally from whom you can learn about crystals. The bear I most often work with lives in the cold North country, in a cave filled with crystals. She is an old grandma bear who loves children and is very patient and protective, as well as playful and strong. If you choose, you can journey to Bear with the specific intention of learning about crystals, and she will spend time teaching you about different crystal formations and their uses. *Power Animal Meditations* has a Journey to Bear that is a good way for beginners to meet her in her crystal cave.

As with the other allies we have considered, the energy of crystals and gemstones can be connected to through their spiritual essence. If you have favorite crystals or jewels you are familiar with on your home altar, you can connect to them from anywhere. You can also call on the essence of quartz, or emerald, or aquamarine, or any other mineral, to work with their specific energies. There are many good books that give insight into the spiritual nature of gems and minerals.

HEALING WITH COLOR

Color has an effect on people, and consequently, can have influence on disease, both physical and emotional.

Some qualitative aspects of color seem obvious—such as blue being cooling and calming, red and orange, warming and active. People who can read auras can gain lots of information about one's state and even one's future, just by reading the colors. To read auras well, however, requires taking into consideration that when you are looking at another's aura, you are necessarily looking through your own first, and if yours is not clear, it will affect the hue of the aura that you are observing.

I also have some concern about the consistency of written tables that codify colors as appropriate to specific organs, illnesses, and so forth. Different parts of our body require different energies at times, due to the circumstances of the moment. It seems to me that our color needs are changeable and very much related to the elements and the colors one would associate with the elements.

Following is a journey that provides an opportunity to learn more about color through connecting directly with the spirit of the color. Once you have taken this journey, you can access color in this way. Or use the journey to learn about the qualities associated with specific colors and apply that knowledge in your healing work.

Sometimes you can play with the water and it will give you rainbows. You can ask about specific hues and about mixing colors as well. Every time you come to this sacred spring you will be given a teaching that will further your knowledge about color and how to use it in your healings or in other artistic practice.

★ ☽ ★

JOURNEY WITH COLOR

Prepare yourself as you would to take a sacred journey. . . . Use the abbreviated cauldron alchemy to come into the presence of Thoth. He is dressed completely in white and is standing beside a stream, which gurgles sweetly over polished stones between an open meadow and a forest of ancient cedar trees. He is holding a white robe that is meant for you to put on once you've purified yourself in the cold, clear water. When you are thus prepared, Thoth leads you as you follow the course of the stream to its source, a small pond fed by a sacred spring pouring from an opening in an out-cropping of large, round boulders with impatiens blooming from the crevices between. A small waterfall casts a spray through which a rainbow dances as the sunlight sparkles upon it. . . .

There is a sense of enchantment here, as though you are in a place between the worlds, where magic lives. Thoth motions for you to reach into the water. Cup your hands together and dip into the sparkling water. As you scoop the water from the pond, it is a clear, transparent color in its absolute purity. Whatever color you have received will have a teaching for you. . . .

When your experience is complete, take off the white robe that has been covering you, and hand it to Thoth. In that moment, as you return to your physical form, you become aware of colors that you would not normally have noticed in your own body. You can only see them for a brief instant, during which you are given an insight about your physical body, or your mental or emotional state.

Ground and center. . . .

12
HEALING TECHNIQUES

FOUR RULES

Because Alchemical Healing is an art form, I'm really not much into rules. The ones I do suggest are important for safety in any healing activity.

When practicing Alchemical Healing, once you have established a connection with the spirit of the disease or injury, you usually attempt to draw off the pain, toxin, or trauma by pulling it out of the body with your hand or hands. Here is where the four rules come in.

1. *Always, when you take anything out of a person you must give it somewhere to go.*
   Illness can be understood as spirit requiring awareness. Once you become aware of the spirit of the disease or the aspect of the problem that can be removed, there are ways to simply take it out. Sometimes the spirit literally jumps out and into the palm of your hand while you are working. In Alchemical Healing the healer is responsible for conducting the energies

that are being manipulated. For example, if a person has a broken leg, you will encounter pain, trauma, and swelling as particular attributes of the condition you are facing. We will be discussing a variety of skillful ways to approach and remove each of these attributes.

As you learn to remove unwanted energies, pain, trauma, tumors, or whatever, it is important for you to respect the energies and to conduct them in an appropriate manner to a place where they can be transformed into their next level of potential. I usually conduct energies that I remove into the earth, and always with a prayer for their transformation into their highest potential. When you are first learning, it is important to gather the energy in both hands, carrying this bundle of energy away from the body of the person to where you can direct it into the earth. It doesn't matter at all whether you are on the ground, on a first floor, or high up in a high-rise building. You simply direct the energy with your intention, pointing your hands toward the ground.

Why the earth? The earth is where our debris is transformed into nourishment. If you are working with particularly virulent energies, you might choose to use water as a medium to hold and transport the spirit energies. First directing the energies into a container of water, you can then release the water at the base of a large tree from which you have asked and received permission. The tree will work with the energies and help in their transformation process. You can also release that water into a moving watercourse or river, or into the ocean or other large body of water. If none of these are available, you can bury it in the earth, again with a prayer for its transformation into its highest potential. If you choose to use this method, be sure to cover or seal the container and keep it out of reach of children and animals if there is a gap between the time when you draw out the energies and the time when you release the water.

In doing this, it is important to remember that no energy is intrinsically bad—unwanted perhaps, even dangerous, certainly inappropriate to our good health—but not bad. Working in a nonjudgmental way, the healer is able to help not only the healee but also the spirit of the energy that is being removed. For example, when a person has a tumor and it is determined that it is time for the tumor to be removed, as a healer you attempt, with your skill, to achieve resonance with the frequency of the tumor—with its vibration and energy. It is a kind of communication, and when you have achieved it you can begin to coax the spirit of the tumor out of the body. Once the spirit leaves, the tumor, the physical material mass, will have to disintegrate. It is just the same as when a body dies; the spirit leaves, and the physical form decays. And since you have conducted the spirit of the tumor into your chosen medium and prayed for its transformation, you have helped to move it forward in its evolutionary process. Our illnesses are our teachers, and we need to honor and respect them.

2. *Never take anything out of a person without refilling the void.*
   Neglecting to refill leaves a vacuum into which unwanted energies can enter. This is a very important rule. Empty spaces will be filled—it is the nature of reality. As long as you are taking responsibility for this work, it is best to see that those spaces are filled with intentional, helpful, and healing energies. Always start and end with the Universal Life Force. To that you can consciously add your intention and other energetic remedies appropriate to the health condition. You can use whatever healing energies you conceive of that have practical applications for the specific situation. Remember, you cannot lavish too much Universal Live Force into a person; he or she will simply stop receiving it once enough has been received.

3. *If you make an opening in a person's field, you must close it.*
   Whenever you make an opening in a person's energetic field,

such as when you are performing a psychic surgery, you must close and seal that place of opening throughout the auric fields of the person. Every person has an aura that extends out from his or her physical body. There are a number of levels, called fields, that are close in, and you can feel them with your hands.

Try holding your hands above the body, at about eighteen inches away. Feel for an energetic connection to the person from this distance. Now slowly begin to move your hands closer to the person's body. If you move in increments, you will notice that you can feel different layers.

When closing the auric fields after a psychic incision, it is important to continue the movement of bringing your hands together throughout each field, starting just above the body to about three feet or more from the body. (More detailed instructions are given in Chapter 16, "Advanced Healing Techniques") This rule applies to any form of opening that you might employ, such as the laser cut or the sucking cure. It is unacceptable and impolite to leave someone walking around with a gaping hole in his or her auric field.

If a person comes to you who has had medical surgery, chances are his energetic field is still open. Surgeons are very good at stitching up the body, but are not aware of the openings they leave in their patients' auric fields. You can find the openings by scanning with your hands at various increments out from the body. Sometimes you can feel the energy escaping. Simply by consciously bringing your hands together, palm to palm, you can close these gaping holes. If you are with someone who is recuperating from surgery, try this and notice whether his healing happens more quickly than expected.

If a person has had a lot of trauma, or drug or alcohol abuse, she is likely to have holes in her aura as well. You can actually feel the openings from which the energy is leaking. I find my left hand more sensitive to receiving this kind of information, so I move it slowly over the outer field, about a foot or so from the body, using the eyes in my palms and fingertips to sense the change. Sometimes it feels like a chill, or a slight breeze or movement outward. Again, close the holes by bringing your hands together palm to palm over them.

4. *Always remember to disconnect.*
At the end of every healing, it is important to disconnect, to separate yourself from the energies you've been conducting. You have been working very intimately with the person, and your energies have been enmeshed. Disconnecting is a matter of safety for both you and the person you are working with. Skipping this part can result in continued draining of your personal energy. Always thank your guides, the elements, and whoever showed up to help, prior to separating. There are several ways to disconnect:

- You can simply brush your hands together and then blow on them with intention. That will immediately break the connection and disperse the energy.
- You can wash your hands with intention.
- You can create your own ritual of separation, making sure that you are separated from the person with whom you have been working.

THE ART OF REMOVING DISEASE

There are many techniques to assist you in taking out unwanted energies, pain, infections, swelling, tumors, or whatever you feel needs to be removed. Sometimes when you are transmitting energy into a person, you begin to sense a reversal of the energies. That's when the spirit of the disease, pain, or trauma within the area where you are sending the energy spontaneously begins to move and come out into your hands. Although it can be subtle, the feeling is quite clear if you are looking for it. I feel it as a twinge on the eye in the palm of my hand, but some describe it as a current of energy moving into their hands, even as they are generating energy out. It is important to know how to respond when it happens spontaneously, and when you are ready, how to actively and intentionally remove the unwanted energies. Often such an energy reversal is a signal that it is appropriate to remove some of the problematic aspects of an injury or disease. I have found a number of effective methods to use in both spontaneous or intentional extractions.

MAKING A MAGNET

As I have said, my left hand is naturally more receptive, and that receptivity has been enhanced by initiation into the electromagnetic current that increases the drawing potential of my left hand and the generating capacities of my right hand. If you have an opportunity to receive the electromagnetic initiation from an Alchemical Healing teacher, it will strengthen the polarity between your two hands and increase the magnetic pull. It will also clear and open a channel that runs from your left hand up your arm, across your shoulders, and down through your right hand. With that channel open you can pull energy out as though you are a lightning rod and run it directly into the earth without danger to your body.

Even if you have not had such an initiation, you may be able to notice, through attention to the practice of working with the life force energy, that each hand functions somewhat differently. You can, with intention, make a magnet of your hand as you hold it over an area of concern. This technique can be very strong, and I highly recommend it, although it is important to be clear in remembering to gather up what you withdraw and offer it to the earth. You might be going after pain, or trauma, or toxins. If you have connected with the spirit of a tumor, wart, or whatever it is that is causing the problem, you can sometimes get it to relinquish its hold just by tugging gently as though your hand is a magnet. I hold my hand fairly steady; however, as I pull I'm often turning my hand slowly in a counterclockwise motion. I might also pull, then release, pull, then release, all just with tension, like playing a fish. As I pull I can feel the resistance—there is a particular tension that I am working with—and I can feel when something that I am going after, or a part of that, yields and releases into my hand. As I mentioned earlier, my personal signal is a kind of twinge that is usually felt simultaneously by both parties. You will benefit by keeping open communication with the person you are working on, so that you can corroborate the experience.

I immediately take hold of that energy, usually with both hands, and conduct it into the earth, following the first rule of Alchemical Healing. I will continue to draw out, usually in increments, for as long as I can feel energy releasing. At any time during this process I may switch to a different method of removing energies. After two or three passes in this way, my intention turns to refilling the place from which I have been drawing out. I always start with both hands, directing the basic Universal Life Force as I begin to refill the area, fulfilling the second rule of Alchemical Healing. As you become comfortable with this method of working, you will enhance this process with all sorts of adjunctive procedures, such as adding herbs, elements, colors, or other ingredients to fill the void created by the removal. Again, always complete with a lavish amount of the Universal Life Force.

★ ☽ ★

Following is a brief example of this work and its speed and efficiency. Kalita Todd is an Alchemical Healing instructor in Northern California. She relates:

> I ran into a friend in town who had severely twisted her ankle about an hour before. Although I had an appointment to get to, I took a moment to use the magnetic force to remove the energy in her ankle that held pain, trauma, and frustration. I asked her to breathe directly into her ankle and release the pain and trauma with her out breath, into my hands. The swelling and redness immediately disappeared, causing her to exclaim in amazement. I, too, was surprised at how quickly we were getting visible results. I refilled her ankle with pure healing energy.

Her pain was greatly reduced and she was able to put her full weight on her foot. I encouraged her to go home and elevate her foot, and ice it. She recovered very quickly.

I had a similar accident in Egypt last year. I was rushing around the Luxor market helping some of the women in my group with their shopping, when I misjudged the height of a street curb and came crashing down on my ankle, my whole body rolling out into the street. Seeing that I was hurt, a number of men instantly surrounded me, eager to help. They gently assisted me up and onto a stool someone put under me, still in the street. This was a market street, with little car traffic but plenty of helpful merchants. My associate, Kathryn Ravenwood, appeared and asked for some ice, but she didn't wait even a minute to administer it to me alchemically, using the element Water and her intention. The called-for ice appeared quickly, as did an elastic bandage and a taxi to take me back to our boat. Meanwhile, my ankle began changing colors immediately, and blew up with a baseball-sized protrusion that looked as though it was preparing to pop. My future on the tour flashed in front of my eyes, and it wasn't pretty. I determined to work with Kathryn to make sure that I could continue leading the tour, although by the look of things I wasn't so sure. While still in the street, she worked for about ten minutes, using her receptive energy to draw out as much of the trauma and swelling as possible, and calling in the spirit of healing herbs such as arnica and comfrey to fill the space.

When we arrived back at our cruise ship the doctor examined the injured foot to determine whether it was broken. He could not be sure without an X ray, so insisted I stay off my feet the following day. This was very hard for me, as the group was heading off to the West Bank to visit the tombs and mortuary temples. Kathryn continued to work on it when I got to my room, and miraculously, by morning it had lost most of its swelling. I did stay off of it most of the day, but by evening, I was back in town taking care of business. The captain was quite shocked to see me arrive back on the boat for dinner. After examining it, he wanted to know what I had done, as he had never seen such rapid healing. I thought it might be difficult to explain, so I opened his hands and showed him how the energy works. He was a sensitive man and could feel it quite strongly. I look forward to seeing him again when I return to Egypt to see if he has done his homework!

THE STRING CHEESE METHOD

Earlier I spoke of aka, the Hawaiian word for the etheric material upon which our thoughts ride, or the threads that make the cords that connect us and create the tapestry of life. The pain and toxins that we remove from the body attach to aka in their energetic form. When you pay close attention, you can feel it. You can reach in with your little finger and catch hold of a strand or cord of aka and pull it out as if it were stringy cheese, spinning it out with your thumb and fingers. Or simply pull it out like a long thread, subtle and fine like spider's silk. If you use this technique, you must hold it away from the body with one hand and reach down to the origin of the threads with the other, then use your fingers to gather the aka that you are removing. You might even feel it appropriate to snip off the stringy connection to the person's body with your fingers. You may be able to see it or feel it or know its presence as you gather it up and, as always, conduct it into the earth with your prayer for its transformation into its highest potential.

BEAMS FROM YOUR FINGERTIPS

When you direct the light from your fingertips it can be felt or seen as palpable beams that you can direct as extensions of your finger-tips, reaching into the person's body and loosening and/or collecting whatever you are trying to remove. Thus the offending material can be scooped or pulled out and dealt with as in the preceding meth-ods. You will also notice that you can extend your consciousness into the person's body. When the eyes in the palms of your hands have been opened, you can see or become informed through the energy that extends off your fingertips as you focus deeper and deeper into the body of the person you are working on.

CREATING INSTRUMENTS

I have used various instruments, designed and created in my mind or given to me by one of my allies, as tools to get at some things that pose difficulties. For example, I have created a curette device to enter and scrape the womb or other place that may need careful cleaning. I also create tools for efficiency, such as drainage tubes, splints, and cushions.

Some years ago, just as I was completing my radiation therapy for breast cancer, I traveled to Canada to teach at a women's gathering. It was there that I met Anugama. She approached me with a request for healing for a broken back that had occurred four years prior. It was an unusual situation because the fracture was spiritually based. It had happened during a magical encounter with a Mongolian shaman in a forest in Finland, a psychic attack after which she had to be airlifted to Germany for surgery. She had been in excruciating pain ever since. Although I was exhausted from my own healing journey, I consented to seeing what I could do.

Upon engaging the energy, it became immediately apparent that this was something I did not want to mesh too closely with, so I was grateful when a Tibetan *nagpa,* or spiritual teacher, appeared to assist me, through my friend and close associate Chris Tice. The nagpa gave me an instrument with which to extract whatever it was that had been inserted into Anugama's spine; then he took the object from me to dispense with in his own way. It was an unusual circumstance, the results of which were so dramatic as to change the course of my own life. My soon-to-be friend received instant relief and has been free of the back pain for more than twelve years. In the meantime, we began to work together and she opened for me her communities in both Germany and Switzerland in which I've continued to share my work.

In that instance, the instrument was given to me by a spirit guide. When I wish to create something such as a drainage tube, I simply raise my hand, palm facing up, and ask for what I need. If I was working on someone with swollen knees, for example, I might want to create a channel to and opening at the bottom of his or her foot.

I would then reach up and ask for a drainage tube, of a material that would not be abrasive to the person's skin, and that would dissolve back into the ethers from whence it came when its job is complete. I would then wait for the feeling of solidity in my hand and attach the newly created tube to the sole of the foot to begin the drainage into the earth. The person on the receiving end usually describes the sensation of liquid flowing.

Building a drain is common practice. When you do it, don't forget to program its disintegration by saying silently, "when your job is done, you may return back to the element from which you came." This is especially important if you are working in a session and need the process to continue after you are no longer with the person. Using this kind of technique, I have created temporary shunts, pillows to put in between vertebrae to give pain relief, internal splints and poultices, and whatever practical ideas came into my mind at the moment of need. Remember the four rules, and make sure they are incorporated in this aspect of your healing practice. If you leave a drain to continue after you've gone, then you must also provide a conduit that ensures the refilling of the area that is being drained.

REMOVING WITH THE HELP OF TOTEM ALLIES

Power animals and other allies can assist in removing diseases or unwanted energies. When you are aware of your healing work in the context of teamwork, then the member of the team with the best tools for the occasion can be called upon, or will show up. I usually look around for who is in the forefront, and if no one appears, I just do the work myself. However, if the problem is tricky, I ask Thoth to direct me to an ally that would be better for the job at hand. As you form relationships with the elements and allies, you will learn their attributes and the unique qualities they bring to any healing situation. You will then be able to call upon the most appropriate ally from your own experience and knowledge. There are a number of stories related throughout this book that give examples of working with totems in this way.

COMMUNICATION AND SENSITIVITY

Once you have explored these healing techniques and have a sense of how it feels to extract disease, pain, and trauma, you will find a measure of comfort in the process. You will, if you pay attention, feel the movement of the energies and the release of whatever you are withdrawing into your hand. Sometimes it feels as though you are holding a magnet over sand. Did you ever see how the iron particles fly up and adhere to the magnet? That's how it feels. And if you feel it, the person you are working on is also likely to feel the same thing—even if you are on the phone, miles or even continents apart.

Communication with the people you are working on is very helpful. If you can feel it, so can they; and if they feel it, it is more likely that their body will believe and respond on the physical level. Many people see pictures more readily than they feel these procedures, and others need to use their imagination. It is important to note that it matters less *how* one perceives than *that* one perceives. The more senses a person applies to the process, the more powerful the experience, and the more likely that person is to have a direct physical result.

When I am first connecting with a person, I ask her to let me know when she can feel my hands. Many think I am touching them when my hands are actually above their bodies. When I am connected and starting to pull, I ask them what it feels like. If I am working with the spirit of herbs or elements, I also encourage feedback on what that feels like. If I'm introducing a totem or other archetype as an ally, I take the communications to another level—inviting people to share the perceptions of all their senses with me, and encouraging them to begin to make relationships of their own.

For example, I worked on a student in Switzerland who, during the course of the demonstration, was visited by a small, blue songbird who entered his body and flapped its wings all around his heart. It then perched on his shoulder and sang into his ear. When the bird was using its wings like a fan, I asked him what he was experiencing. He said he felt his heart become lighter. When the bird sang to him, a big tear welled in his eye, and he said that he would never have to be alone again.

It is important to establish how the person you are working with perceives the energy. Some may be forthcoming with information about the images that come to them, or perhaps they will hear or smell the experience. With practice you will easily be able to translate their experience into practical guidance for your own creative participation in the process.

There are other viable signals such as images and messages that you might receive while connected with the person through the energy. It is best to encourage people to give you information rather than tell them yours; however, all information that comes to you is useful in determining the direction you will take.

One's sensitivities to this part of the work are cultivated through repetition and practice. It is very much like learning a new language, and it is very individual. As I have mentioned, I am not one who sees pictures. I feel what is happening mostly through the eyes in the palms of my hands. I feel in twinges and tingles and electric impulses, as well as temperature changes and other subtle and not so subtle variances. Only through persistent experimentation do you begin to trust the signals that you get. But once you start to see the patterns, you will find them to be very reliable.

Regardless of which method you use to remove unwanted energies, when you are unable to regain the connection that is apparent within the tension between your hand and the person's body, you have removed as much as you can for the moment.

HEALING CRISIS

There is a phenomenon that occurs on occasion that needs to be addressed. *Healing crisis*—the intensification of symptoms, which may or may not suggest the climactic finish of a disease or problem. This often appears to be a worsening of symptoms. A nagging pain suddenly becomes acute, a swollen sore suddenly comes to a head; it's as if the problem has lived its full life in a short, intense period of time. This is another thing that you can only learn to recognize through experience. It happens often enough that I feel safe to say, you will encounter it. Worsening symptoms, of course, are not always a healing crisis. It is important to be able to discern whether you have a reached a healing crisis or have chosen the wrong technique.

Marie was a student in one of my healing classes. She suffered from a chronic condition of a Bartholin gland cyst. In the past, when it had become inflamed, it had to be lanced. It became particularly swollen and painful during class, so I decided to work with her for a demonstration. When I directed the energy toward the gland, the pain began to intensify and her condition was becoming intolerable. She had to leave the room and go to the bathroom, where she discovered that the cyst had opened and begun to drain on its own, relieving the problem.

DISTANT HEALING

Although when you are first starting out it is best to practice the healing techniques up close and personal, distant healing is as simple as knowing that whatever you do energetically can be accomplished just as easily from far away as it can when you are physically present. Space, and to a certain extent time, are modulated by intention. The easiest way to realize this is to try it in a controlled way. I find the telephone a most useful tool. If you talk someone through the same healing procedures over the telephone, you will find identical responses as if they were present with you in the same room.

Hold your hands out as though your palms are directly over the place you are intending to send the energy. Imagine that the person is right there with you. Sometimes it helps to work with your eyes closed, especially the first few times you try this. As you set your intention and make your Fire Mist Shower, using your power word, do your best to envision the person as though he or she were there with you. If you only know the person's name, that is enough to make a clear connection. If the person is someone that you do not know at all, such as a victim of an accident you have passed on a highway, simply use your focus and intention to connect, and you will feel when that connection is made. (For a discussion on the appropriateness of working on someone without their knowledge, see Chapter 13, "Ethics in Healing.")

Then you can follow the energy as you would in any healing, moving slowly enough to feel each aspect of the work. When you are doing distant healing work on someone with whom you have no communication, you are on your own to feel and know each part of the process as you do it. When you are in communication, you can receive useful feedback throughout the process. As in any healing, the more the person can be directed to feel and see the experience, the stronger the outcome will be.

Any aspect of the healing work can be accomplished from a distance. Often I will work with a power animal or a plant spirit for a person. When I am working this way at a distance, I send the animal or plant with instructions. Sometimes I send it and let its own intelligence direct its actions. If I am in contact with the recipient, I will introduce him to the ally and request that he ask the ally for its help. It's important to get a person to see or feel or simply know the work that the ally is doing. Again, engaging the recipient in the healing process and in providing feedback on the work adds to its potency.

My first experience of distant healing was with a friend who was in a motorcycle accident. Dick was pretty banged up, but the only actual fracture was located in his collarbone, which just required immobility. He telephoned me from his hospital bed. We started with the most peripheral wounds and worked our way into the more difficult ones, the punctured ear drum and the bleeding blood vessel in his head. He would tell me about each problem and I would work there, then we would go on to the next one. He had such confidence in what I was doing and gave me such good feedback that I felt quite comfortable about working at a distance from then on.

It was a few months later that I received a phone call from Lee. She was living in New York at the time, and she was so miserable that she had decided to give it up and take her own life. A mutual acquaintance who was visiting Lee, and who knew of my work, tried to get her to call me, as she knew I was practicing psychic surgery. Lee wasn't interested at first; she had exhausted her resources, tried everything, and was just focused on giving up. Finally her friend offered to pay for the phone call if she would just try, and so I received a call from a very distressed woman in serious pain.

Lee had been injured fifteen years earlier when a horse reared and came down on top of her, crushing a vertebra in her spine. She had been in pain for all those years and had experienced at least one bout with near paralysis. At the time she called, it appeared that she was heading for a wheelchair existence. The calcifications (bone spurs) that had developed were cutting into the nerves that led to her legs, causing severe pain. As the bone spurs grew and put more pressure on the nerves, paralysis was imminent.

Lee is extremely sensitive; in fact she is a medium. When I tuned in to her, she could feel my presence and accurately describe everything I was doing. As I focused on the place of her injury, my intention was to find and dissolve the calcium deposits. That was not what happened, however.

It is important to realize that the energy we are working with seems to be linked to an intelligence of its own. It cannot be stressed enough that when the eyes in the palms of your hands are open, you begin to *see* from those eyes, and are informed in your own way.

Regardless of my intention, when I focused I became aware of the *feeling* of a nerve connected to the palm of my hand. The feeling was very clear, and I interpreted it to mean that I was connected to a nerve that passed through the spinal column at the distressed vertebra. The nerve *felt* like a rusted, corroded car battery cable. It was so obvious that I instinctively began to run pure energy from the tips of my fingers, directed up and down the nerve with the intention to clean and polish it. The result was immediate. Lee said the pain stopped instantly and that the numbing pins and needles turned into the tingling that comes when a body part that has been asleep begins to wake up. We were both quite startled. We stayed with the process until it was evident that a real change had occurred.

I had the impression that in order to keep the nerve protected we would need to do further work. I built a sheath around it and then created little air pillows to put in between the vertebrae to take the pressure off the injured disk. Lee was elated. For a short while she was absolutely free of pain—the first time in fifteen years. Even though this freedom from pain could not be sustained over the long term, it was enough to renew her hope and will to live.

I encourage you to be willing to try anything, no matter how impossible it seems. After all, whatever we do can only support and enhance whatever healing is available to a person if that is our intention.

For another approach to distant healing, try putting your hands together in the *mudra* of prayer, palm to palm. Make the Fire Mist Shower. Begin to pull your hands apart, little by little, feeling the space between fill with the vibrant life force energy. Keep pulling and playing the energy until you have a ball of energy about the size of a party balloon. Begin to imagine the person to whom you want to send healing within the balloon. *See* that person already healed, active in his or her life in a way that demonstrates that healing. Apply as many senses to the image as you can, imbue it with more of the Universal Live Force from your hands, and when it has become fully clear and complete, use your power word and toss the balloon upward, releasing all attachment to it. Be sure to immediately turn your attention elsewhere, so that your newly created thought form will find its own way into actualization.

MULTIPLE HEALINGS

Another interesting effect I have noticed with the energy is that although you may be directing it to a particular person, with a specific purpose, it can be picked up and utilized by anyone aware of or within the energy's field of influence.

One day a friend came over for a treatment on his back. He was in considerable pain and I used a form of psychic surgery to enter his back and create an etheric splint to hold his spine in place. A friend who happened to be visiting at the time witnessed this healing; she was in the same room, about six feet away. After the treatment was complete, she took me aside to relay her astonishment. She had been in a car accident about eight years earlier in which her knee was damaged with an injury that had never completely healed. During the time I had been working on Moz's back, she experienced a spontaneous healing. Her pain was gone, and movement was fully restored.

This experience opened up all sorts of possibilities in my mind. I began to experiment. If I were working on a person at home, I would phone a friend that I knew was injured or sick, and also another, using the conference calling service. I directed the healing to the person I was working on in hopes that it would reach the other two people through the telephone. It worked often enough to validate my observations.

During this period of discovery about multiple healings, I was invited to be interviewed on KPFA radio in Berkeley by the late Will Noffke, who produced a show called "New Horizons." I called Will and told him I wanted to experiment with his audience, but before I could tell him the nature of the experiment, he stopped me short. His show was live, he said, and whatever I wanted to do would best be done on the spur of the moment. He did not want to hear about it until then.

Will was the perfect person to initiate me into radio. His manner and interviewing style put me completely at ease and gave me every opportunity to come across in a positive light. I was so comfortable

talking with him that I forgot what I had decided to do. About half-
way through the hour, Will said casually, "You mentioned you want
to do an experiment. Tell us what it is that you propose." Bang. Just
like that.

"I want to try to heal the audience," I replied with much more
confidence than I felt. Will barely raised an eyebrow as he picked up
the idea with enthusiasm. As I attempted to explain how it worked,
he caught on immediately.

"You mean it's like an extension cord with lots of outlets? You
can plug many things into the same current at once? An iron, a
radio, a TV? I get it." His enthusiasm gave me more confidence.

First we suggested to the audience that if any of them were driving and wanted to participate in the experiment, they should pull
over and park for the moment. I told them to focus on whatever
they wanted to heal, and to pay close attention to the feelings that
came with the energy I'd be directing. Then I proceeded to guide the
audience through a psychic surgical procedure as I performed the
work in the air (and on the air) in the studio. I could feel the magnitude of the force that was coming out of my hands. It was huge. I
told them to pay attention and feel as I made the opening and went
into their bodies. For me it was like entering into a deeper layer of
reality. Then I suggested they keep feeling as I pulled out what
needed to come out, whether it was pain, old trauma, tumors, disease, whatever. During the refilling part it was as though tremendous light was pouring from my hands. Then I closed the incision
and sealed it, and it was done.

The response, through letters and the people who showed up at
Will's center, where I led a workshop, indicated that the experiment
was a major success. More importantly, we were able to understand
and share another dimension of metaphysical law as applied to
healing.

PROTECTION AND EMPATHY

For most people, the processes used in Alchemical Healing are safe and inclusive of protection. The Fire Mist Shower is your first line of defense, along with your awareness. In general, grounding, centering, and making the Fire Mist Shower will activate a protective force field. By acknowledging where you are in relationship to the six directions, you place yourself at the center of the universe and in a position from which you are grounded and secure. If you are attentive to your own inner signals, you will usually know if you have to take further protective measures.

Many healers are empathic. Healing and empathy seem to go together—maybe because the desire to heal comes from the experience of suffering, which fosters compassion. Empathetic people are so sensitive that they can feel the pain of others. This can be quite isolating, for when such a person enters a crowded room, he can pick up so much that it becomes difficult to be around crowds. Such people tend to think that empathy is a curse; however, it is actually a great gift.

Your first shield, and the most important aspect of protection, is your awareness, which is especially vital for empaths. It is through awareness that you can distinguish between your own pain and the pain that belongs to somebody else. Developing your ability to discriminate is an important tool of protection.

Once you understand the nature of being empathic, you can use the information that you receive from your senses to help you as a healer. You can tell not only what and where the problems are, but you can also tell when they have been alleviated.

PROTECTIVE SHIELDS

If you find that you are so sensitive that you need further protection, your next line of defense might be to try creating an elemental shield as described in the exercise below. Many people have problems moving about in the increasingly congested environs of our cities, particularly in shopping malls, while traveling through airports, or when they find themselves in other situations where crowds gather.

EXERCISE

Protection—Creating an Elemental Shield

Start with Earth. Reach up over your head or the head of the person for whom you are building the shield. Draw the yellow square sign of Earth in the air with your Earth fingers, and reach up through the window you have created with both hands, feeling for your connection to the Earth element. As you approach Earth, hold a strong intention for the aspects of Earth that you want to draw down into this shield, and *feel* as you connect to the Earth element and begin to draw it down through the window and around the field of the person or yourself. Pull it around the body, creating an egg-shaped shell of Earth like a net of gold, intended to allow in all positive energies and filter out any harmful ones.

Next, reach up and draw the Water symbol with your thumbs and pull in the Water element with the intention of adding a reflective layer to the shield that will return any unwanted energies, yet allow the desired ones to pass through. Envisioning the reflective layer as a mirror can be helpful.

Fire is next. With intention and by drawing the symbol above the body, create a fiery layer, as though you are surrounded with an egg-shaped covering of Fire that will burn or consume those energies that could cause harm.

Air will surround the body like a feathery cushion that will both protect it and invite humor and lightness into the surrounding field.

All four of the gross elements—Earth, Water, Fire, and Air—should be used when you are creating this type of shield.

Psychic and emotional debris as well as other toxic elements are becoming pervasive. Once you have initiated yourself to the elements (see Chapter 10, "The Elements"), you will find it easy to draw the elements around yourself, or around someone else, to create an elemental shield as a means of protection. This technique is also useful for protecting those who have a tendency toward accidents. The shield requires occasional revitalization, and is much stronger if you create it after the symbols and elements are wired into your hands.

Shields Made by Allies or Totems

One way to ensure your safety is by calling on your own totems or protective allies. Certain animal totems and deities, or other spirit guides, can be guardians and protectors. In your youth and innocence you may have felt the presence of guardian angels or other beings that just happened to be there to pull you out of harm's way. When you have taken steps to become a person of power in your own right, it becomes more your own responsibility to protect yourself and to ask for the help you need. It is suggested that you call on your protective allies and ask for their protection.

For example, I had been told to invoke Anubis—the jackal god of Egypt who is guardian of the underworld—as a protector at each direction when I was traveling in Egypt with my groups. On this particular occasion, I realized I had only remembered him at one direction; but I didn't think much of it. The following day when my friend Chris Tice and I visited the Cairo Museum, we went to commune with Anubis through the exquisite statue of him that guarded the treasury in Tutankhamen's tomb. Both of us could feel rage coming off the statue. This was the only time I ever felt actual anger from one of my major allies. It reminded me in no uncertain terms that I must *always* call on Anubis and ask for his protection from *every* direction when traveling in Egypt. We walked away from the statue somewhat shaken.

Later that afternoon one of the group participants approached me nervously. She told me that she had observed me while I was engaging with Anubis and had respectfully waited until I had left before approaching the statue. Standing in front of Anubis, she felt anger, and wanted to know what it could have meant. I was astonished, and thanked her for telling me, because it was an exclamation point to his message for me. I assured her it was not meant to be taken personally by her. She was relieved, and I was twice reminded.

Now I call on Anubis for protection whenever I head into a strange or difficult situation, and there are others I call on as well. We must never take our allies for granted, and the most valuable gifts we can give to them are our gratitude and our attention.

Most shields that you make for yourself are meant to protect you from common danger, not premeditated attack. Until there is a quantum leap in consciousness throughout our planet, there always will be envy, fear, hatred, greed, and jealousy; and a person of power, especially one who is enjoying life, can become a target. If you are apt to encounter focused and directed negative energies, you can create appropriate protective shields in a variety of ways.

It is important to note, especially if you are dealing with people who have studied or developed personal power, that any shield or method of protection that is written about can be neutralized by a person sharing that knowledge. When I am teaching protection in my classes, I journey the participants to Sekhmet to receive a shield directly from her for each of them individually. That way, no one else can be aware of the shield and it becomes integrated into the person. Often these are living shields and must be kept vital through attention and love.

Our greatest protection besides our awareness is the way we live our lives. Those of us who are committed to change are not hiding under our beds or in our closets; we are out engaging with life, acting in order to fulfill our purpose. Our first responsibility is to ourselves, to take care of our bodies, our minds, and our spirits, and to remain vigilant to what is happening around us at all times.

A NOTE ABOUT TECHNIQUES

Each of the techniques we use in Alchemical Healing is a powerful and effective tool, yet it is always important to remember that the tool is not the most important part of the healing process. Think of techniques as if they are part of a scaffold. When you are constructing a large building, you use scaffolding to support you at the different levels of the construction project. But once the construction is complete, the integrity of the building itself is what holds you up. If you continue to focus on the techniques as the primary healing resource, the scaffold you have built becomes the kind of scaffold that holds a noose or a guillotine.

13
ETHICS IN HEALING

BEING A HEALER DOESN'T REQUIRE a new set of ethics; it requires hypervigilance. It asks you to constantly question your motives while you strive to be completely present to each moment. One does not graduate to superhero status as a healer: if you think you've arrived, it's time to start over. Healing is a humbling experience.

Ethics in healing is a complex topic that brings up many issues. I have tried to cover the most salient points, at least those to which I would hope each person who takes up these tools will give considerable thought.

WHO IS THE "HEALER"?

To understand who is actually doing the healing in Alchemical Healing, one must look at the dynamics of the healing process. A person is in need of healing. That person contracts with someone who has experience with bringing relief and healing, through both skillful means and invoking and working with supportive energies. You now have the person seeking to be healed, the practitioner, and spirit—which includes the allies, elements, plant spirits, and any other sentients that are invoked in the process.

You can't say that any one of those three components alone is the healer; it takes all three aspects engaged in order to make the healer, and to achieve the healing. When the three parts are working together, it is a dance for which there is music, and both human partners, the practitioner and the healing recipient, are integral dancers moving the process. All participants share in directing the process. The practitioner may lead initially, but when the dance is happening in a fluid manner, the leading is transferred from one to another, with all three taking turns. The music for the dance comes from outside of the two people. Music, in this metaphor, is both the magic, and the result of magic. The person being healed gets into the rhythm under the guidance of the practitioner, who has experience both invoking the energies and guiding the person into awareness of them: the "healer" starts the process and brings the person's attention to the music. By actively participating, they are moved by subtle energies that they become aware of as they engage in the process.

The subtle energies are here all the time. It is through the process of forms such as Alchemical Healing that we become aware of them. The person being healed has invited the healer to apply his arts to invoke this process. Meanwhile, these rich resources come into play and have more sway with the physical realities. Who is the healer? The healer is the totality of all involved. The active combination of the healer, the healee, and the allies results in a whole that is greater than the sum of the individual parts.

WHEN DO WE CALL OURSELVES HEALERS?

There are ethics around how we present ourselves, what we say we can do, and who we say we are.

Calling oneself a healer is likely to raise eyebrows in many circles. "Hi, I'm a healer." Instant turnoff. In actuality the process of healing is a joint effort. But as is so often the case, language is inexact, and better alternatives are unavailable. ("Hello, I am an expediter of energy transference between you and what your higher self and the universe have already decided.")

I practiced this work for many years before I felt comfortable with calling myself a healer. I needed to develop not only my confidence, but also my skill, a history of results, and most important, the certainty that I am not doing the healing by myself, no matter what I'm called. I am now comfortable calling myself a healer. I have a track record.

At what point can you, the reader, call yourself a healer, knowing that it makes some people uncomfortable to be confronted with that title?

Ultimately, I can only speak for myself on the question. I avoided the appellation of healer for many years as I was developing mastery of my craft. It sounded arrogant, especially considering the true dynamic of the process. However, eventually, as healing work consumed more and more of my life, and the progress and results of the work lent more confidence to my self-understanding, it became comfortable by default: I couldn't find another good word to describe myself for those who asked.

The day the words "I am a healer," or even "I am a healing practitioner," come out of your mouth, listen to them in all humbleness, knowing that you have *not* crossed a threshold that removes you from constantly standing in awe of the magic. You have not mastered or taken control of the magic, only acknowledged your participation, your willingness to be part of it. Alchemical Healing provides an umbrella under which the art of healing can flourish, as long as the practitioners remain clear about what they know, and what they can do.

I strongly recommend that you make it a rule to avoid promising a specific outcome in healing. If you create expectations that go unfulfilled, it may negate whatever real healing did take place; you can only promise your best efforts. Besides, you can never tell what a specific outcome is going to be, and you always want to leave room for something magical and unexpected to occur, even outside the ordinary framework of time. There is also the danger that if expectations *are* fulfilled you may conclude that *you* have performed a miracle.

MIRACLES

What is a miracle and who performs it?

Miracles are dramatic, extraordinary, often spontaneous healings that occur, and that are beyond the reach of our imaginings. I mentioned the miscarriage that I witnessed miraculously reversed in the presence of the loving spirit of Hippopotamus. The disappearance of cancer before surgery or treatment, the spontaneous mending of broken bones and wounds, the complete disappearance of severe symptoms, the disappearance of burns and swellings, the shrinking and disappearance of tumors: these are other examples of miracles I've witnessed.

We can ask for a miracle, we can be honored to witness a miracle; however, we do not create miracles. Sometimes miracles even happen without our asking.

Many years ago I received a phone call from a mother of a five-year-old girl who was facing surgery for a tumor that had developed on her kidney. It was during a time when I was unable to see the girl directly, so I promised to do a distant healing session before she would have the final tests just prior to surgery. I felt an intuitive desire to work with Thoth on this particular healing, but whenever I went to him he seemed to have another agenda. As the time for her final tests neared, I got concerned and approached Thoth for help yet again. This time when he wished to focus on another subject, I interrupted with my concern for the child. He gave me a severe glance, then lifted his arm and threw a lightening bolt off his fingers in the direction where the girl lived. He then turned back to the lesson at hand.

The following day I called the child's mother and told her the work had been done, although I refused to take any credit for it. I asked her to let me know the outcome of the next round of tests. Some days later, I received a phone call from a very excited mom—the doctors were unable to find any traces of her previous symptoms, and the surgery was called off.

Another miracle of sorts happened when my daughter Sage, at about ten years of age, broke her foot just before a trip to Jamaica. When the X ray confirmed the small fracture, the doctor wanted her to wear a cast, which would have severely limited her freedom to play and swim at the beach. I went to work with the skill I had at the time, and the swelling and pain vanished overnight. She never wore the cast, and has never suffered from any weakness in that foot. Was it my skill, her desire for freedom to swim, or divine intervention? My guess it was all of us together dancing with the magic.

WHAT IS OUR RESPONSIBILITY IN HAVING THE GIFT?

The free will that is an inherent part of human life is a pertinent issue for healers. It is up to the individual healer to determine when, where, how, and why to respond, regardless of the circumstances. We all have response-ability—the ability to respond—according to our skill, experience, and the situation we are faced with.

Insofar as the laws of the land relate to medicine and healing, there are also consequences to our responses that we should look at before we take certain actions. Regardless of how safe we know this work to be, we live in a suit-happy society where issues of malpractice as well as practicing medicine without a license pose real dangers. Another of my occasional rules would be, never offer healing in place of conventional Western medical practices. I am always careful to tell the people that I work on that this alternative healing form is an adjunct to rather than a replacement for traditional medical care. Just because you see a cobra eat a tumor doesn't mean you should abandon the medically prescribed treatment. You still need to validate your subjective experience of healing with objective tests that corroborate your findings.

As to the gift itself, we must all wrestle with questions about our responsibilities. For me, the time for this came at the beginning of my practice of healing, right after receiving the Reiki initiations. I tackled the question of responsibility as a healer, and I have not had to deal with it since. I had just discovered the power of laying on of hands and had completed Reiki II the previous weekend. I was in California, on my way to a Grateful Dead concert when, as we approached the Golden Gate Bridge, a car coming toward us veered into the traffic divider and crashed. We could see the driver's head slump over. I pulled to the side of the road and my brother-in-law, Dicken, jumped out of the car and ran to see if he could help.

At the same time, another car had stopped, this one with a doctor, so Dicken soon returned and we continued on to the concert. I had noticed immediately, when the accident happened, that my hands had lit up and started running energy, without any intention or volition on my part. I simply noticed the process and kept on going.

At the concert, I decided to practice using the dynamic of the audience and music to see how the new Reiki empowerments worked. I had a perfect place to sit, at the front and center of the balcony with no obstructions between the band and myself. It was a great concert, one that happened to be a benefit for some antinuclear causes, and it had the special energy felt only at benefits.

I began to use the Level II Reiki symbols to connect to individuals I knew who were in need of healing. There was the friend in Texas who was in a coma from a failed liver, and several others who came into my mind. I intended my connection with each person, drew the symbol in the air, and felt as that person became connected with the music, the energy coming off my hands, and the energy in the concert hall. I held each one there until I felt solid strength and consistency with the current of energy with which we were connected; then I continued on with the next person. In a sense I was stringing them all together and using the energy of the music and the audience to amplify the energy for healing.

Things were moving quite well until I remembered the man who had been in the accident on the freeway. From a friend at the concert who had passed the scene on the highway a few minutes after we had, I had learned that he was alive; he was wearing a neck brace and entering an ambulance when that friend had passed by. As I began to draw the symbol that would bring him into the healing force that had been created, my mind was suddenly filled with questions that I had not considered before: Who was this person? How do I know when it is okay to offer healing? What if I intervened in his life and as a result he later went on to hurt someone? Would I be responsible in some way? Is a person ever not deserving of healing?

The bright, colorful, celebratory scene around me turned a dull gray. I found myself retreating into an introverted, self-absorbed funk, which did nothing for me, nor for any of the people I was trying to help. The questions swirled around in my head, spiraling into a confusion that, when I finally had the presence to ask for clarity, gave way into a clear, sweet knowing: for me, the gift of healing asked only for open-handed generosity, with no obligations. The gift was neither to be withheld nor forced, and the choice would always be mine based not in blanket judgments, but in the clear determination of appropriateness in the moment.

Having the ability to help relieve the suffering of others is a gift-that comes with response-ability, the ability to respond. It is with great humility that I give thanks every day for this gift, for it truly does keep on giving.

PERMISSION

There are varying opinions among healers as to whether or not you need permission to send healing to another person without that person's knowledge. I have been told by some that one should never direct healing to a person without being asked. I have also been asked to send distant healing to people that have no way of asking. And, as in the situation described above, I have had my hands turn on without volition in the presence of need. I don't believe there is a hard and fast rule that gives a final answer to the question of permission, although good manners might be a good place to start. When possible, ask. When not, use your intuition and your common sense. If you find yourself spontaneously responding to suffering, whether coming upon the scene of an accident or while watching the evening news, it could be an empathetic resonance. This is a non-verbal form of communication that, according to some, is equal to permission. Part of you responds to needs around you without thinking about it. Do you just witness or do you consciously participate? Personally, I rarely stop to think about it if I have a strong urge to direct energy. My commitment to the universe is to help whenever I can, and I view this response as doing just that.

What does one do when asked to work on a third party who has neither asked for help, nor given permission? It could be someone in a coma, or perhaps a child who could not make such a decision. It could be a stranger you just read about or a friend or relative. I am of the mind to go for it. I trust that the universe will convey somehow the need to stop if I'm trespassing. I also know that the subtle energies we are directing can be employed differently than is our intention, or can simply not be received, but I am content with the efforts made. Some others in our field wouldn't dream of volunteering energy where not specifically requested. Employ the wisdom of your High Self in every situation. Recently I received a phone call from a woman that I don't know personally, asking me to pray for her son who was facing an imminent court date. I had no qualms committing to and complying with her request. How would you have responded? If you have trouble concluding for yourself, you can always defer to your High Self, journey to Thoth for guidance, or consult the person's High Self. Many people create dialogue with the High Self of the person in question, and offer their energy to be used in accordance with the will of the recipient. It should be noted that when a person has granted permission, they are also agreeing to engage in the process at some level, which is always helpful.

PRIVACY

The same ethics of patient/client privilege that doctors give their patients should be afforded your clients in Alchemical Healing. Information you learn through your work is private, and not to be shared with others without express permission. It is also important to remember that you do not need to know personal details that are brought up during the journeys. Often people will want to share, but they need to know that they have the choice. Even when they are faced with remembering childhood traumas or past-life tragedies, it is not necessary for you to know the details in order to guide them appropriately. And if you do know those details, it is important to remain objective, confidential, and nonjudgmental.

Another thing: you should never give someone's name and say, "this is what I did for him." Your stories are part of your history, and sharing can be inspiring to others. But think of your healing experiences as sacred, a part of your sacred history, shared with respect and honesty, yet never violating the privacy of those involved. (For this book I've kept to nonspecific references or first names [some changed] except where permission has been granted.)

REMUNERATION, RECIPROCITY

When I was developing my craft, I was eager to practice and engaged with enthusiasm at every opportunity, with no thought of compensation, monetary or otherwise. It was, and often still is, enough to engage in the process and hone my abilities with every new experience. Also, I have a hard time being around people who are suffering without offering to do something about it, if I am able and if they are open to the possibilities.

There came a time when my financial needs, my strenuous schedule, my guidance, and my sense of confidence all conspired to move me into a more professional relationship with the healing work I was already practicing. The argument that first served to support that transition was the idea that I could charge for my time, even though I might find it difficult to charge for the essentially free gift of energies that spring from an infinite source and flow through the work. As I became more proficient, skill also became a consideration.

It has gotten easier for me to distinguish when to charge and when to give away, especially since I began to recognize that energy spent in the service of healing comes back to me in other, often surprising ways. It is of primary concern, however, that whatever arrangement has been made is honored. It is equally important that you not bring your personal needs into the healer/client relationship. As a healer, you must take on the task of doing your own work around money and abundance. Doing that work allows you to enter into healer/client relationships with integrity and grace.

If you are indeed fascinated with transformation, then you will be less tempted to look to your clients primarily as a source of income. On the other hand, few of us have the luxury of being taken care of in a way that allows the full-time generosity of carrying the mantle of healer without reciprocation. And, too, reciprocation has its own intrinsic value. In Alchemical Healing, clients are generally involved in their healing process. Involvement has its own merit. Consequently, they get benefit partially in accordance with the value they assign to the work. Those who haven't made a reciprocal offering sometimes make less progress in their healing.

In many of the old tribal cultures, a person would go to the healer or shaman who is responsible for the ongoing health of the tribe. The person desiring the healing would bring firewood, food from her garden, cloth, tools, or other desirable commodities. In our culture of industry and technology, where most people no longer grow vegetables or weave fabrics, the currency for trading has changed from goods and services to currency of another sort—the green energy that is money.

Paying somebody money in our material world is an act of commitment. It is important to have commitment from those to whom you offer healing. Having a clear contract with monetary remuneration is certainly a way of obtaining that commitment.

It is easier for a client to place value on your healing work if you place a value on it yourself. If there is to be an exchange of energy, whether in the form of money, trade, or barter, it should be clear at the outset of the work. Vagaries only cause problems after the fact. Integrity implies honesty and openness; therefore, it is common sense to make clear with your clients what the arrangement is in regard to payment. Whenever possible, it helps to consider the lifestyle of the person. Sometimes a situation is a time for charity; and it is always a time for generosity.

COMPENSATION AS AN ASPECT OF RECIPROCITY

In Peru, the Quechua society, which predates the Incas, hold as most important to their way of life the concept of *ayne*, the Quechua word that can be translated as *reciprocity*. Every gift received and every action taken is part of a complex code that is expressed in their *despachos,* their agreements with one another, and their ceremonies. Many Native American tribes celebrate the *giveaway* as an essential part of their code of conduct, especially in honoring the gifts of vision in ceremony, gifts of healing, and gifts of learning.

These customs recognize the truth that in order to remain expansive, or simply to keep growing, each of us must constantly empty our cup to make room to receive anew, whether it is new teachings, new understandings, or new material stuff. Aspects of this truth are meaningful to both the healer and the healee.

Reciprocation can manifest as some sort of tithe in gratitude for the gifts from both humans and spirit. Often it is as simple as remembering and making offerings. As a healer you are responsible to the teachers and the spirits that help you, and must always honor and credit the source of your teachings. This can be as basic as remembering with gratitude as you explain what you are doing while working on someone, or buying groceries for your elders, or supporting their projects. To disrespect the source from which the teachings come is to disrespect the medicine you are passing on in your healing work. If you don't value the source, it will have no value; you will shortchange the process.

BLENDING TRADITIONS

Many ancient tribal traditions are falling away because the children who would naturally have inherited the knowledge are giving up their roots and moving from remote areas into the distractions of city life and urban survival. Often the seekers who find and learn from various indigenous elders mix and blend the teachings, rendering it difficult to distinguish specific cultural or traditional lines. This also tends to water down the original knowledge.

Because Alchemical Healing is in and of itself an amalgam, it would be a difficult exercise to separate the sources of the knowledge; however, the form is consistent and maintains its own integrity. I have walked a number of roads in my sacred journey of Alchemical Healing. The sacred Pipe and the ancient Egyptian spiritual paths may appear to the casual observer to be polar opposites. Actually, there are many similarities. When I am walking the Red Road with my Cannunpa, I adhere to the rules as they were given to me, for it is not up to me to change them. To do so would compromise the tradition as it is being handed down, and would subvert my own objective of honoring and preserving these wonderful traditional ways.

On the other hand, I am well aware that all spiritual paths are alive and require some spontaneity to keep from degrading into dogma and rote, the bane of religion. There are differences between religion and spirituality. Religion requires the organization of beliefs and often the structuring of ritual. This generally aims at a consistency that is important, but it engenders a loss of vitality as prescribed liturgy becomes rote. Spirituality, on the other hand, is expressive of the moment and the active relationship between the practitioner and spirit.

I suggest that if you are combining formal traditions in your spiritual practice or working with traditions that are struggling to maintain their integrity, you weave these traditions carefully. It's like braiding hair. If you take up three portions of hair and bring them together into a braid, the beauty and strength of the braid is in direct relation to how well you keep the integrity of each of the plaits, separate and honored unto itself.

WHAT TO DO WHEN IT DOESN'T WORK

As you pay attention to your work as a healer, you will see that each healing can proceed in unexpected ways. Your own desires and preconceptions are often irrelevant, and the open-heartedness required applies to the entire healing process. This can be particularly difficult in circumstances when someone is suffering or near death, because the desire is often to relieve someone's suffering or keep him from dying.

We must be open to the possibility that the pain or even death is inevitable, regardless of our wishes. The presence of pain and the threat of death are obvious indications that healing is called for; however, you must remain clear about whether healing or intervention is appropriate in this particular moment and circumstance. Ultimately, you have to trust yourself.

You may have to accept and forgive yourself if, because you want the person to live, you are too emotionally distraught to be clear. Perhaps the best thing you can do at a time like that is to recommend someone else who is less emotionally involved, someone who can hold the space for the lessons that are present even in pain and in death. We are growing, evolving beings, and there are times when we are not clear, during which our hearts are not open to the will of spirit. If you feel the need, help your client or beloved find someone who will do the necessary work with an open heart. Yet remember, there can be no harm done when you offer the Universal Life Force to any person, anytime. Your intention can be as simple as to offer up the energy to be used in accordance with the highest outcome for the person, whatever that might be.

What happens when it becomes obvious that you are not helping your client? Inevitably you will experience healings during which you are stymied; you cannot get a response from your client and you do not know where to go next. When this happens, it is important to stay calm and to refrain from placing judgments on either yourself or your client. Sometimes, it is simply not a good match. Know where the resources are in your community so that you can make appropriate referrals to get the person to the practitioner that is right for him.

★ ☽ ★

Sometimes you might find that you have entered a domain that is over your head; perhaps you discover that you are doing damage to your client that you didn't expect. The most frightening experience I had during a healing happened in front of 150 people during a demonstration at a conference in London.

A woman asked me if I would work on her husband, who was in great need. I was in a hurry at that moment, so I told her to bring him to my lecture and I would use him for a demonstration. I neglected to find out what the problem was. When it came time for the demonstration, I invited him to come forward and asked him to describe his situation. Apparently he was suffering from stroke-like symptoms, although there was no evidence that a stroke had taken place. He was able to articulate clearly, and I assumed that the source was in the wiring of his brain's nervous system.

He was sitting in a chair facing forward, toward the audience, and I was standing behind him. I placed my hands over his head in order to make my initial connection. Then I put my attention in my left hand and began moving it around slowly, feeling for information. Immediately I felt a strong and very specific sensation in the palm of my hand, the sensation I associate with nerves. It was *quite* strong, and I gently maneuvered my hand to attempt to get more information.

Because I was so keenly focused, I was not aware of the audience at first, but I sensed emotion rising in the room. I paused and looked up to see the audience moving to the edge of their chairs, some covering their faces with their hands. I wasn't sure what was happening, so I positioned myself so that I could see what they were looking at, and when I moved my hand the slightest bit, the man's face contorted with the movement. I stopped moving and asked him what he was feeling. He opened his mouth to speak, but no words came out. The audience gasped, and I was suddenly gripped with fear.

Inside, it was all I could do to keep from panicking, for of course I knew that I had to stay calm. I knew that the answer was available to me, and that I had to maintain my center. I held quite still and took a deep breath, then called on all my allies and helpers. I opened myself up and asked Sekhmet to come inside me so that her keen sensitivities would find the appropriate response. I allowed the allies to do the work, and I waited quietly while that was happening, trusting in the process and knowing that even if I could not see or hear or feel what was being done, it was happening. After a few suspenseful moments, I asked him again, and this time, to all of our great relief, he could speak.

Sometimes we have to step aside and trust in the alchemical process, and often, as was the case in this demonstration, we healers have something to learn or remember. The lesson for me was clearly about getting out of the way and trusting. In terms of ethics, I have always considered that it is vital to leave the person in at least as good condition as when they came to you—and that can take some doing! The man I worked on in the demonstration didn't necessarily make great progress, however, he was not harmed.

Another example of when it's time to give it up happened during the construction of our home. One of the carpenters cut off the tip of his finger while moving a heavy wooden hatch cover onto a fifty-five-gallon drum. I washed the wound and the finger tip, then put it back in place on the end of the finger and held it there for a few minutes with intention to adhere. When I took my hand away, the fingertip was sticking to my hand instead of his—we took him to the hospital immediately and the fingertip was reattached with no problems.

PERSONAL ACCOUNTABILITY AND BOUNDARIES

I cannot stress enough the fundamental importance of personal accountability in healing. It is probably the most important aspect of ethics. Always remember, you are accountable for everything you say and do, and any advice you choose to give.

It is especially important to remember that Alchemical Healing is an adjunctive form when working with clients who are already in treatments such as radiation and chemotherapy, or any of the accepted treatments for AIDS and other serious afflictions. You *must* be respectful of other forms of treatment, and work with harmony and cooperation in mind. No matter how well a person seems to have responded to a healing, results must be checked, and the tests that are afforded by Western medicine are invaluable for monitoring purposes.

You must also be accountable, as stated earlier, in the sense of completing whatever work you start in a way that leaves the person in at least as good shape as when you began. It is better to say no when it is appropriate to say no rather than to abort a session in the middle, without bringing the work to a suitable conclusion.

As a healer, especially if you get very skilled at your craft and garner some notoriety, you must have boundaries. You will need to establish limits on your time and how much you are willing to give. It is always good to err on the generous side, but you also have to be careful to keep from being sucked dry, or you won't be good for anyone. It is in the nature of those that are called to this work to want to give selflessly, and our natural inclination is to be generous. Your health and strength are vital to the continuance of the work, so be clear in your boundaries.

Although I never like to turn a person away on the basis of money, I have established boundaries between what is free and what is included in a fee. Sometimes I get called a lot, for support or for having my brain picked. Having a clear policy is helpful, even though some flexibility is advisable.

Ethics in healing, as in any other vocation, is a personal standard that each person must develop and fine-tune for him- or herself. I hope these rough ethical guidelines and stories from my own experience will be helpful to you.

PART III

ADVANCED ALCHEMICAL HEALING

14
THE CADUCEUS

ELEPHANTINE ISLAND IS NAMED for the huge boulders that encircle its southern end, hard gray granite boulders sculpted and rounded by the rise and fall of the Nile through the millennia. When I take my groups to Egypt, we sail to the island by felucca, small sailing boats manned by smiling Nubians who sing and drum while ferrying us across the river from Aswan, the southernmost and most picturesque city in Egypt. Aswan is nestled at the foot of what used to be the cataracts that separated ancient Egypt from the lands to the south, before the building of the old Aswan dam and the more recent High dam. The ancient Egyptians of the north thought that these cataracts were the source of the Nile, and that the god Khnum determined the inundation, the yearly flood that brought new life to the parched lands of Egypt.

Temples were erected on Elephantine many thousands of years ago, dedicated to the god Khnum and his consort Satet. It is believed that the Ark of the Covenant spent time here, possibly in an ancient synagogue that has been located in the midst of recent excavations. Of all the sites we visit in Egypt, Elephantine shows most clearly that Egyptian temples are layered, one on top of another. The late 1990s saw the opening of an area of the excavation that allows us to enter a newly opened temple beneath a more recent one, heightening the sense of walking back through time.

I prefer to do ritual at the top, in the courtyard of what used to be the ancient temple dedicated to Khnum, a ram-headed god who creates the physical form of humans out of clay on his potter's wheel. Although the temple has been reduced to rubble, with only an entryway left standing, it is the perfect place to work on grounding— grounding ourselves in Egypt, connecting with the land and her energies, and opening and clearing the circuits in our bodies. It is here that Thoth confers the caduceus, his staff of power and balance.

The caduceus is an example of a Greek symbol sourced in Egypt that lives prominently in our Western mainstream culture, primarily as a logo representing medical practitioners and companies involved in healthcare. The American Medical Association is the most well-known group to use it. Each part of the image has a meaning that, when it comes alive in a person, creates enduring changes.

The principle power comes from the two snakes that wind their way up the central staff, the spinal column. The two snakes represent the kundalini energies that move up the two etheric channels which, in Eastern (Sanskrit) lore, are called the *ida* and *pingala*. These are the conduits that carry the energies of the earth up through the body so that they can unite with the energies brought down from above, bringing the physical and spiritual realms together. Serpent energy rising in a person's body is the same as the kundalini energy seen in the Eastern imagery. The snakes of the caduceus are associated with the elements Water and Fire, female and male, yin and yang.

The central staff is the spinal column, the *shushumna* canal, the primary channel for our energy. To the ancient Egyptians it would have been the *djed* pillar, the backbone of Osiris. The staff appears to be made of metal, perhaps gold, and represents the element Earth. The wings of the caduceus represent Air, the element that we associate with our higher self, that aspect of our self that connects us with spirit. These wings unite us with the entire cosmos and give us

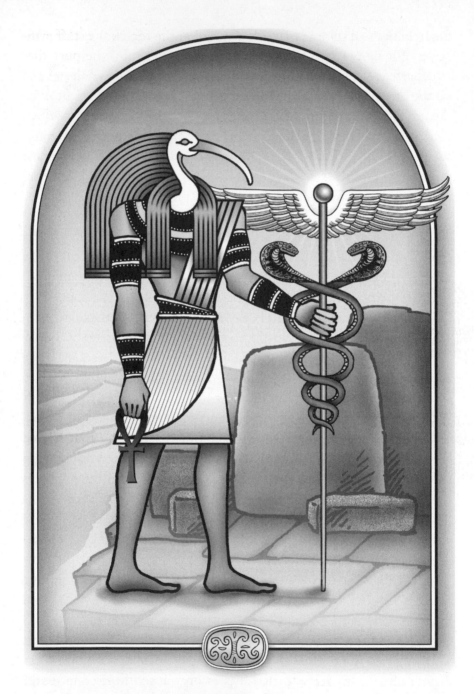

Figure 14.1. The Caduceus

the freedom to explore it. The round ball at the top of the staff symbolizes both the prima materia, (the first matter) and the pure diamond body, the essence of spirit. It is superimposed over the pineal gland, in the center of the brain, and is pictured as a glowing crystal or diamond orb. Occasionally it appears as a pinecone, for which the pineal gland was named, perhaps because of the similarity in shape. This may well be the stone, the first matter, which, when infused with spirit, is transformed into the diamond body, the universal medicine, the philosophers' stone.

Together these symbols express optimum balance and the connection we all have to higher cosmic intelligence. When you meditate on the caduceus, it ignites currents of energy in your body, giving a boost of energy not only to the physical body, but to whatever activity, healing state, or visualization you are working on. As a practice, meditating on this symbol will confer balance, inspiration, healing, and the ability to accomplish your goals. It will also serve to maintain clear and vibrant channels through which source energy can flow through your body and out your hands and fingers for healing, if you so wish to direct it.

People need access to energy beyond their personal stores if they wish to heal others: they need the electromagnetic field that source energy provides. When one receives the opening to the life energy that the caduceus empowerment provides, the life energy carries with it an electromagnetic field. When the energy increases, the electromagnetic field increases. At this time on earth, people need more energy and require a stronger electromagnetic field. The earth's magnetic field is currently decreasing. Without intervention, our individual fields will also decrease. When greater volumes of energy become present in people, the energy itself eventually teaches people, at its own pace. It brings healing, at its own pace.

The following caduceus empowerment provides the foundation for any serious practitioner of Alchemical Healing. This process includes the basic elements of preparation for any healing practice: gaining access to the infinite source of the Universal Life Force, activating the third eye, and connecting with Cobra, one of the most powerful healing allies. It is recommended that you enter into this journey as a meditation practice on a daily basis. Obviously, reawakening the caduceus every time you practice healing will prove greatly beneficial. Refreshing this empowerment will become quick and smooth and will continue to teach and transform with each new experience. Eventually, it is hoped that practitioners will maintain a level of balance and clarity that is sustainable.

INITIATION

CADUCEUS EMPOWERMENT

The first time you do this journey, you should be standing if possible. Prepare as you would for any major initiation in this book, making your space sacred, smudging yourself, and invoking your allies.

Close your eyes, relax, and take some deep breaths. Ground and center. . . . Do the alchemy that brings you into the presence of Thoth. . . .

You are standing on the stone foundation of an ancient island temple, surrounded by the flowing waters of the Nile. Thoth stands before you, carrying his staff of power, the caduceus. Two cobras entwine around a central rod, with a crystal or diamond orb at the top and wings that extend to the sides. It is a powerful and graceful symbol of balance, and he holds it toward you so that you can see it clearly. . . . Take a moment to familiarize yourself with the elements of this staff. . . .

He touches it to your body, and you feel the central staff enter and merge with your spinal column. Notice how your back naturally straightens. . . .

Direct your attention downward, into the earth beneath your feet. First become aware of the layers and layers of sacred space, where temples were built upon temples, each giving renewed consecration to this powerful vortex. . . . Now you become aware

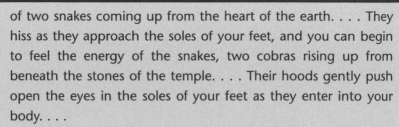

of two snakes coming up from the heart of the earth. . . . They hiss as they approach the soles of your feet, and you can begin to feel the energy of the snakes, two cobras rising up from beneath the stones of the temple. . . . Their hoods gently push open the eyes in the soles of your feet as they enter into your body. . . .

Allow yourself to feel as well as see, imagine, or simply know their presence as they slither their way up through the central meridians in your feet and legs. Notice the sensual way in which they move up through your body, cleansing and clearing, coming together and crossing at the first chakra center at the base of your spine, igniting and spinning the glowing center at the root of your being. . . .

Take a deep breath and as you inhale, be aware of the cobras as they continue winding upward around the staff of your spine to the second chakra. As they slide upward, awakening every cell, they are followed by a flood of golden light energy, purifying all in its path as it pours through you. . . . Exhale, as the cobras intersect at the second chakra. . . .

There is an opening and clearing as each chakra and channel fills with liquid light energy as the cobras course upward. All blockages melt as the energy increases in intensity. Inhale again as the cobras wind their way up toward the third chakra, then exhale as they intersect through the third center at your solar plexus. . . . You may feel a pulsing as the third center ignites. . . . Take another breath, as though you are inhaling the snakes upward. . . . As you exhale, the snakes move into your heart center, where they stop for a moment to bask in the radiance created when the liquid fire they carry mingles with your radiant heart fire. . . . Another breath and they move upward, their scales vibrating against your chest as they wind toward your throat. . . .

Once they have opened your throat chakra, they enter your head and now move, carefully, up through the inside of your head to behind your eyes. They pause, the energy pulsing. . . .

Allow them to look through your eyes. . . . What do they see when they look through your eyes?

Now they will let you look through their eyes. . . . Stay with your new vision for a moment, until you have retrieved the perspective they wished to show you. . . .

The cobras move up through your crown and turn their faces upward toward the sky. . . . They hiss, and their hiss is like a call. . . .

From a far distant source, from deep within the center of the universe, the response comes as a rain of grace, the pouring down of a fine spiritual energy. . . . It enters your body through your crown and also pours down around you, making everything it touches tingle, every cell and molecule, until it is as though you are standing within a shower of shimmering energy. . . .

The cobras move back into your head and take their place on either side of your pineal gland. . . .

Now place your attention on your shoulder blades, and you will feel your wings begin to sprout and fill with this refined spiritual light. You have beautiful feathers of light, rippling with the subtlest of movements, filling with energy. This light comes pouring down your arms and hands. . . .

Your arms lift and extend as you feel your wings stretch out from your sides.

Take a moment to scan your body and feel what it is like to be in the balance of the caduceus, the energies of earth and sky united within. Notice how the power moves through you. . . .

Put your attention once more on Thoth. He now holds a crystal or diamond sphere, which he shows to you before he places it in your third eye. . . . It enters and goes to the top of the staff, surrounding the pineal gland. As the energies raining down from above and coursing up along the staff from below intersect in the orb, there is a dazzling explosion of light. . . Gradually your inner sight clarifies. (To an observer it would appear as though your heart flame has been refined through the lens of the sphere, and a lavender glow is rising out of the top of your head.)

Hold your attention in the fullness of this experience, as the essence of joy and the power of love permeate the whole of your being. . . .

Become aware of how grounded you are, and center yourself in the balance that this initiation has conferred. . . . Before opening your eyes, stay with the feelings that have been aroused in you for some time in order to integrate your experience. . . .

The Caduceus Empowerment is complete for the moment. There is much more evolution that will come from practice. The balance and power conferred will strengthen and become more consistent as you integrate and retrain your body and spirit through practice over time. The more you do it, the more naturally it lives in you.

RESULTS OF THE CADUCEUS PRACTICE OVER TIME

From Danielle Hoffman:

> I always do the Caduceus Empowerment before working with people. One of the gifts from this empowerment is the balance and protection I receive from the practice. I have a tendency to be a little sponge-like and take on other people's energy. With the caduceus activated in me, I come from a place of power and balance that transforms my vibration from sticky to whole and complete. There is no space to take on other people's stuff—for me a great blessing.
>
> The Caduceus as a practice has also provided me with a daily

ritual to deepen my relationship with Thoth, the cobras, and the winged ones. It has helped me come to recognize their signature energy, especially the winged ones that change from day to day. I can feel the difference between Nekhbet and Thoth wings, or the crow or Horus. This has helped me to hone my sensitivities beyond the sometimes nebulous identity that I think of as Thoth, to recognize his signature no matter what form he shows up in. The cobras are also invaluable in healing sessions. The caduceus gives a foundation for me to study directly with Thoth and for him to teach me ways of healing that I don't think would have been possible without the discipline of greeting him each day. Through this practice we have come to understand each other's language and expressions.

As a kundalini yoga instructor I have found the caduceus an effective and quick way to raise kundalini energy and to keep these channels open. The cobras come in and cross at the sacrum where the kundalini is stored. When ignited, it rises with the snakes in the ida and pingala and up the central channel of the spine, almost as if there is a third snake or as if the staff that Thoth places in the spine becomes alive in this kundalini essence. I often have a vibrating sensation in my body.

From Bo Clark:

For me the caduceus brought a place of peace, maybe the missing link, into my work. It is an integral part of my life. It comes without being called upon when it is most desperately needed for assistance with healing at global proportions. It has brought a peace and calmness within that shows up when I am involved in healing work. It has taught me to get out of my own way and trust that it is all for the higher good, whatever the outcome, and to not be attached to that outcome. And it leaves a place for the work and the healings to evolve at their own designated pace, and as always, leaving room and space for the magic to happen!

Because I am part of this lineage, I began to incorporate the

Caduceus Empowerment into my own classes. I saw and felt shifts in myself and in those I was working with, both in classes and in healing sessions. A calmness and confidence moved within me, and Thoth became even more discernable as a co-creator of transformation. I watched as he moved among the students, unbeknown to them, and I saw the students move more readily into acceptance of who they are and who they can be. I saw many students who seemed disconnected but interested in the work, while still searching for a niche to fit into, actually sway and shift and emotionally feel the caduceus grow within their own bodies and deepen their relationship with Thoth. They felt its strength and power and accepted it with openness and honor. Many expressed amazement as they came to understand the gift that was being given to them.

From Kalita Todd:

In my experience the opening of the channel of the Universal Life Force is the basic tool of many spiritual paths. I had learned to open this channel in other ways; however, using the form I have learned through my apprenticeship with Nicki has taken this ability to a whole new level of usefulness and enhanced my capabilities. Visualizing the snakes coming through my body makes this energy flow clear, powerful, and tangible, and when needed, the opening can be instantaneous.

In my own life and healing work I practice the Caduceus Empowerment almost every day, often in the morning, or any time I am inspired by music or nature or when help is needed in the form of healing work. This practice helps me to stay grounded and centered, and to experience life more fully awake and available. It adds a sweet richness, for I never feel alone—I always feel cared for and connected to a greater whole. As the meditation develops I find myself standing in a column of light that begins to filter slowly down through my body. It is deeply relaxing and feels as if all my parts are being set into alignment, culminating when sky and earth have united in my body. My spirit guide, Thoth, stands before me and touches my third eye. Beginning at my first chakra, a tantric wave of energy begins, which builds until all chakras are open and streaming with energy. All that doesn't serve the highest good is shaken off. When this undulating wave dies down, my guides are there to greet me. They often speak to me as we stand in circle together, ready to start the day.

COBRA AS A HEALING ALLY

The energies of Cobra are a vital part of the Caduceus Empowerment, and their presence in your life, especially if you are doing healing work, brings the juice, the joy, and the wisdom into the body. Whereas Thoth brings you the mind and the intellect, Cobra *feels,* and conveys the wisdom of the earth and of your physical body. Hence, she is a potent ally worthy of your wholehearted attention.

Cobra is a powerful symbol in Egypt. Known as the great awakener, Cobra appears on the crown of pharaoh as the guardian of Lower Egypt, the delta lands of the north. From her seat on the uraeus crown (the circlet adorned with the cobra goddess Uadjet that was worn on the brow of pharaoh) she would spit fire at his enemies. Many goddesses have cobra aspects, and even Thoth can appear as a cobra in the underworld. Consider the feathered serpent of the Aztec, Quetzalcoatl, another example of corresponding energies in diverse cultures.

It is important to develop strong relationships with your cobras. They are potent healing allies, with tremendous wisdom to share. As a part of your healing team, Cobra is ever present (especially if you practice the caduceus!). Cobras, being all spine, are particularly effective when you are working with back problems. They have very different systems than we do and can devour many diseases because they are not vulnerable to the same pathogens as we are. And they love to eat tumors.

Once your caduceus is in place, Cobra is right there to whisper in your ear and offer suggestions about any healing you do. She travels easily through your body when you have problems. You can send one of your own cobras to work with clients, or simply summon another to appear. Sometimes Cobra might spontaneously emerge through the palms of your hands or anywhere within your internal view to participate in the work in progress.

What is key about working with Cobra, as with any totem or ally, is attention: the attention you give, and the attention that the person who is receiving the healing gives. Attention is the coin of the realms. Attention is what you pay—and what you pay is in direct proportion to what returns. So it is important to apply all of your senses toward perceiving just what the cobra is doing. If she is eating a tumor, the person being worked on must feel and hear and use all her senses so that her body will know that the tumor or cells or virus or whatever is actually being devoured.

When I first started working with Cobra in the late 1980s, I did not tell the people I was working on about her. I was afraid that she would frighten them. I can still remember the first time Cobra took over during a psychic surgery. I was sitting in a friend's living room with Dave, a man who had come to me to try to find out what all this "new age metaphysics and healing" was about. I had a hard time articulating what I was doing because we didn't speak the same language. I suggested he tell me about some malady he experienced so I could show him by demonstrating a healing. At that, he lifted his shirt and showed me an infected cyst that protruded from his side. He had been seeing a doctor and was taking antibiotics.

I started to work on him, using my hands above the cyst, but not touching it. I felt an extremely strong connection, and he was right there with me, attentive, though quite surprised to feel the subtle energy connection so strongly. As I was preparing to enter into his body using an energetic laser technique that would give me access to the cyst and the opportunity to remove it, I became aware of Cobra. In my mind I asked her if she was hungry—perhaps she would like some lunch? I sensed her affirmative response and told her to go for it. I could perceive her lightning swift movement as she darted her head into his body and took the spirit of the cyst in one gulp. I said nothing about it to Dave. But when I attempted to connect to the cyst that was still physically in his body, I could not feel a thing. My work was complete; there was nothing left for me to do but lavish energy into the area.

Although the demonstration took barely a moment, Dave had clearly felt the initial connection, and his interest was piqued. The next morning when he woke up, he discovered that the cyst had completely disappeared. Stunned, he called me immediately. I was too shy to tell him about Cobra at that time, although I did start teaching about her in my classes. And the more I worked with her, the more I realized what an important ally she is. When I finally did get up the nerve to introduce her to my clients, most were easily able to recognize her and invite her to help with the work.

Eventually I recognized how important it is to engage the person's attention in whatever is going on as much as possible during any healing process. The more levels on which a person concurs with what is happening, the more likely he is to respond fully to what you're doing. If you are working with any ally, every sense applied increases the internal belief system. In the case of Dave's cyst, it didn't matter. This was a small cyst and I could tell in the moment that its removal was successful. But in many situations, it is apparent that the job will not be completed in that one sitting. In those cases I give clients the suggestion to continue to work with Cobra every day. If they pay close attention, if they can feel or see Cobra actually eating the spirit of their tumor or disease, their bodies will respond in kind. Their deep attention is vital to this part of the work. If the spirit is removed, then the physical manifestation *must* disintegrate. The disappearance of matter when spirit vanishes follows a basic natural law. It is also important, however, to use this method *adjunctive* to whatever treatment they are already undergoing.

MORE COBRA STORIES

Cobras can be very powerful allies for healing spinal problems, especially with regard to flexibility issues. I once had a student whose son was a member of a prominent ballet company. This young man had sustained a debilitating spinal injury that forced him to quit dancing during the time needed for recuperation, and after a year or so he was convinced that he would never dance professionally again. His mother asked me to work with him, and during the one session we had together, Cobra appeared. I suggested he make eye contact and open his heart to this ally and ask for her help. As soon as he made clear that she was welcome, she entered his body and worked her way down his spine, as though she were blending her body with his spinal cord. There she stayed for quite some time, long after our session was over, reminding his spine of its innate flexibility. It was not much later that this talented young man was able to return to his professional dancing career.

Richard was a doctor who came on one of my tours to Egypt. The night before we were to travel to Aswan where we were to board our cruise ship for six nights on the Nile, I got a call that he needed to talk with me. He was distressed because a kidney stone that he had been aware of suddenly became inflamed, and he was in serious pain. He was concerned that it would require medical attention while we were on the Nile, far from any hospital facilities that could handle his needs, and that perhaps he should leave the tour before such an emergency occurred. I could not really assure him of another outcome, and told him that he should do whatever he thought best under the circumstances. I did suggest that he had nothing to lose by letting me try to deal with it first, and he could make up his mind in the morning before we left.

I had never before attempted to remove a kidney stone and had no plan when I began the work. I made my connection and felt the source of his pain quite strongly in my hands. As I held my hands over his kidneys, I received a distinct impression that Cobra was there and wanted to assist. I told him a little about Cobra and asked him to bring her into his awareness. Then I guided him to greet her, make eye contact, and open his heart to her while asking if she would be able to help with, or might enjoy eating, his kidney stone.

Richard was able to perceive the cobra quite clearly as she entered his body through the urethra. He could feel her as she moved up through his bladder and finally into his kidney, where she proceeded to munch the stone, then depart from his body and coil at his feet with a satisfied expression. He offered her thanks and went back to his room somewhat bewildered from the experience, yet quite willing to allow the stone to disappear. We agreed that he would determine what to do the next morning.

Richard never experienced the presence of the stone again—it simply vanished. We had a fabulous time for the rest of the tour.

★ ☽ ★

Often Cobra works in mysterious ways. Following is a story in the words of the recipient of a healing given by me some years ago. From Nancy W., Mar 29, 2000:

> I was having serious bleeding problems with a fibroid tumor on which my doctor said she couldn't operate because of its location. You were gracious to allow me to be used for demonstration in one of your Alchemical Healing classes on March 7, 1999 in San Francisco. I took the Cobra energy inside of me and you told me to continue to work with it on my own. I agreed. The bleeding got a lot worse, and in desperation I demanded to see my doctor in person to discuss alternatives. She took one look, got excited, and said I was dilated and "giving birth" to my fibroid. That was a Wednesday afternoon (April 14); she scheduled surgery for Friday morning, during which all she had to do was to snip the cord that had formed. My doctor was very impressed and even more so when in a follow-up exam I told her I had gone to a spiritual healer. (I didn't go into details about the cobra energy.) I certainly consider the resolution a miracle, as does my doctor. I didn't know what to do with the cobra afterwards, so I just thanked it and released it.

Kalita Todd, an Alchemical Healing teacher in Northern California, had this experience working with her mother:

> My mother was diagnosed with colon cancer that had metasta-sized into her lymph nodes. She changed her diet, started a regimen of vitamins and supplements, and began a series of low-dosage chemotherapy treatments.
>
> I worked with her alchemically by introducing and assisting her in creating a personal relationship with Cobra. Since the cancer could migrate to anywhere in her body, the visualization I offered her was that baby cobra snakes would enter at her feet, eat all that didn't serve her highest health, then move on up into the ankles, calves, etc. She was instructed to send her breath into each area as it was being worked on. As the snakes left an area of the body cleansed, that area would turn green, a color that can represent healing. She was to continue with this visualization until her entire body was a healing, green color. This exercise also helped her to relax deeply and she was then able to sleep soundly.
>
> My mother told me of the deep concern and fear she experienced when she went for her chemotherapy treatments, especially while this toxic substance was entering her body. I suggested that she call on the snakes and ask them to meet the chemicals as they entered, to direct them to where they needed to go to do the job of destroying cancer cells, to witness as the chemicals did their work, and then to eat the residue. This visualization empowered her to participate in her own healing and use the dangerous yet powerfully effective chemotherapy to her best advantage.
>
> My mother went into remission during her chemotherapy series. She never lost her hair and only experienced an infrequent loss of energy. She resumed gardening and square dancing before she completed her treatments.

Three years later she received all good reports and the cancer is still in remission.

15
AKASHA

AKASHA IS THE MEDIUM from which all of the elements are derived. As the matrix of the creation, Akasha holds patterns of information in the same way that the night sky holds constellations, in a multidimensional grid that is the home of consciousness as well as the origin of the material forms we see in our world and our bodies. It is the macrocosmic spiritual mirror of our DNA, which is the microcosmic blueprint of who we are. Each of us has our individual blueprint, the design underlying our being, which fits into the matrix of a cultural and racial collective. Consciousness permeates this blueprint as it permeates the whole of creation. Our evolution is concerned with the comprehension of consciousness, so that we as a species can participate in our development in ways that are more co-creative and aware.

One needs a foundation of experience in the other four elements before working with Akasha. Moving directly into work with Akasha would be like running a marathon before you learned to crawl. The tricky part is simply retaining presence while working with this etheric substance. It takes considerable practice just to stay awake, and power is lost if you sleep through it.

When you learn to hold your attention and focus in the dimension of Akasha, the *in-potentia* reality, you take an active, conscious role in the act of creation. Akasha, by whatever name or language, is the domain of avatars. Those who sustain full clarity and presence here have the opportunity to achieve mastery.

Energy follows thought, and thought precedes form. We struggle to control our thoughts and often race to catch up with the senseless spinning of our minds and our random daydreaming. Many disciplines such as Rinzai Zen Buddhism, Vipassana, and other forms of meditation, yoga, and martial arts can help us to develop some control and focus, to quiet the constant chatter, and to develop our concentration. When we fully honor the power of our thoughts, it becomes a priority to train our mind in a conscious and beneficent way. We have to develop the power to sustain constant presence, to concentrate, to be clear in our intention, and to honor our experience no matter what is happening around us and no matter how we are challenged. If we remain vigilant, we will function at a higher level where we can be consistently informed through Akasha.

Because Akasha has the attributes of a spiritual or universal solvent, it is easy to lose consciousness and feel yourself slipping off to sleep until you become accustomed to working in that realm. In some systems this element is referred to as *ether*. Although *ether* now brings to mind a gas used as an anesthesia during surgery, Aristotle used the term to explain where you go when you leave this three-dimensional realm. It was thought of as the substance in which the planets were suspended.

Thoughts have power. Pure thought is amorphous and is not measurable. As thought is consciously held, Akasha forms itself around it to create the initial blueprint or pattern for its manifestation. This pattern attracts the other elements required to bring it into form. These elements come out of flux, out of the solution of Akasha. As each molecule is added, reformed, or combined, this three-dimensional grid becomes the matrix for the new manifestation. It starts to build substance, and as soon as the elements congregate around the pattern with sufficient mass and energy, physical manifestation occurs.

There is also great power in the spoken word. Putting a thought into words concretizes the thought and brings it even closer to manifestation.

To work successfully with Akasha for either manifesting or healing, your thoughts need to be very clear. Chatter, doubt, and inner conflict siphon off energy from a portion of your creative potential. If any of these mental states are present, you either won't get what you are intending, or the results will be distorted. To intentionally manifest with Akasha, hold clear, purposeful thoughts with loving energy. If you feel yourself begin to drift, you must come back to clarity with grace and gratitude. Don't give yourself a hard time; it only compounds the problem.

HEALING THROUGH TIME

Clear, loving thought assists in creating something as simple as the manifest well-being of a person who is sick, or as complex as the blueprint for a new bodily organ. Although Akasha allows us to view past and future as well as present, it is more about presence than about time.

If you were using Akasha to rebuild a damaged liver, you would also engage the aspect of Akasha that holds all time as simultaneous. In this circumstance you would use a combination of Earth and Akasha to go back through time to remember the original pattern of health and wholeness within the liver *before* it became diseased. You do this by drawing on Akasha in increments, each time first drawing in Akasha, then holding and grounding in Earth. As you hold Akasha with the appropriate intention, you are informing the body of the original blueprint at the time of your focus.

Keep track of how many times you draw Akasha until you have found the original pattern of health that existed before the disease began or the injury occurred. Once you are holding that original blueprint, keep your focus and continue drawing Akasha while you reiterate your intention and use your power word to enhance the process. As the original healthy image is brought to the foreground, the healthy pattern emerges. The elements needed to bring this pattern into form are attracted to the pattern, and the cells begin to be restructured. Each cell has its intelligence and starts taking responsibility for its immediate area. If this pattern is overlaid on the area of the damaged liver, the things that don't belong, like scar tissue and toxicity, go back into solution and flow away. What you are left with is the healthy liver that the body remembers and recognizes rather than the damaged one.

EXAMPLES

Gayle was on her way to one of my classes when she was in a car accident that totaled her car. A friend picked her up from the hospital and brought her to where the class was taking place. I went to work on her immediately, using the opportunity for a demonstration in the use of Akasha.

I started by working with the techniques of basic Alchemical Healing, directing energy into her body and removing trauma wherever I found it. Her principle injury was to her knee, which had become quite stiff and swollen and very painful. I pulled out as much of the pain as I could and put in soothing and healing herbal spirits. Using the technique described above, I drew on Akasha, and went back to before the accident, easily finding the pattern of health that existed before the injury. I held the space for the pattern to shift to the original healthy one, then brought that pattern back through time to the present. The immediate result was the return of movement to the knee joint and the lessening of pain.

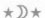

A friend was suffering from depression that was quite debilitating. She had retreated inward; she found it difficult to communicate with her family and had almost no contact with others in her circle of friends. She was a good friend of mine, and I respectfully allowed her to process in her own way and in her own time. Although she had been seeing a therapist for some time, she finally asked for my help one day while I was visiting. I asked her if she was willing to be healed instantly, rather than dragging it out. When she said she was ready to have the depression gone, I went to work, calling on Akasha to permeate her being. I asked her to remember a time before the depression set in, a time when she felt good about herself and what was happening in her life. While that information was coming in, I started working back with Akasha, and grounding it in Earth. When I reached a place where she felt self-confident and energetic, with no sign of the depression that held her in its grip, I poured still more Akasha into her, and used my power word. We stayed with that initial experience in which she found her healthiest emotional patterns for a few moments, and then alternated again, grounding in Earth and working with Akasha while moving back through time to the present. We also moved forward in time using the same process to anchor the new pattern of healthy responses to the parts of her life that she thought might be influencing her depression. By the end of the process, her depression had completely lifted. On her next visit, her therapist corroborated the change that happened.

The following story is about the first healing I did on my husband, Mark Hallert. He had been injured in the Army in 1969 and had had two subsequent surgeries. For this healing I used the technique described above. I will share the story in his words:

> It was a good day—my knee didn't hurt. As I approached Nicki's house I didn't need my cane. I walked in, set down my bags, and leaned my cane behind the door. Nicki called me upstairs. She had heard that I had been having trouble with my knee lately and offered to work on it. I so badly wanted this healing to work. Not because my knee was bothering me so much, but because I was very attracted to Nicki and I wanted to be a good subject for her healing arts.
>
> Fast-forward a couple of hours. My knee was driving me crazy. I couldn't figure it out, this combination of itching and burning and being oversensitive. I dropped my pants to see what

was happening. There was nothing visibly wrong—and then it hit me: For the first time in fourteen years since the first knee operation, I could feel the skin on my kneecap—it was the denim rubbing on the newly sensitized skin that was driving me crazy.

The cane has gathered dust for many years. It's still sitting behind the door.

AKASHA AND DNA

Our DNA is the physical manifestation of the blueprint that is built in Akasha. In our lives we respond according to the information patterns encoded in our DNA. Our bodies take their shapes and characteristics from it, our behavior patterns are in direct relation to it, and our DNA patterns are passed on through us to our progeny. How much of who we are and what we make of ourselves is genetically or environmentally based? That question has been pondered and researched and debated, with no final answer. Yet we know that we can change things, even fundamental characteristics. As explained earlier, we know, too, that if we alter the basic patterning or blueprint of a living thing, a direct result appears in the physical world.

DNA is a governing device that helps us to make order from chaos. The DNA assures that each cell knows its own role. At the same time, each cell shares the same DNA code that informs the whole body. Whether it is bone, corpuscle, or sinew, Akasha calls upon its perfected state as it would exist without environmental or biological damage. With your focus and assistance, you can overwhelm the pathogens with healthy cells by using Akasha (rather than DNA) to inform and revitalize the cells in the body.

All of the information of the ancestry of an individual is encoded in our DNA. There is no beginning and no end in this realm. It is conveyed to us through the interaction of Akasha and consciousness. Our awareness of that which is contained in the DNA spiral at any given moment gives substance to reality and gives us the illusion that we understand our material world, helping us to avoid the madness that would ensue without a higher level of order encoded in the patterning. DNA is the information base, the foundation that gives us the confidence to face chaos in a largely uncertain or at least unknown universe. It is a marvelous mystery that we can be grateful for.

At a certain point it is up to us to consciously offer back to the spiral of DNA information the wisdom gleaned from our experiences, thereby contributing to a more conscious evolutionary process.

I used to think it was a shame that we made our contribution to the gene pool before we gained our wisdom. Now I see a way we can contribute to the gene pool as teachers and guides for the youth who have yet to procreate. As our knowledge and experience accumulates, we can add to the collective DNA our personal experience and wisdom through the intentional and focused use of Akasha. There are at least two ways that we can do this:

1. We can pass wisdom on as allegorical stories, fairy tales, poetry, and literature. Wisdom can be expressed through music, dance, and other arts. It must be offered in such a way that the youngsters who receive this wisdom can take it into the essence of their being and be moved by it. It is the responsibility of elders to make our stories alive so that they catalyze insight and realization that is then added to the coding within the DNA.

2. We can also acquire and pass on wisdom through magical acts and rituals that use the fundamental principles of Alchemical Healing. When steeped in Akasha, the intention for these practices will be recorded in the records of each of our souls, our DNA and Akashic Records. This honoring results in subtle alteration of the collective DNA, and conscious evolution of our species. Wisdom itself cannot be learned from another. Information can be taken in, but only experience can transform it into wisdom. And no matter how smart you are, if you don't pick up the tools you have when you need them, your will to accomplish will come to nothing.

THE AKASHIC RECORD

If the DNA is like a scientific filing system that contains the body's knowledge, then Akasha is like a computer hard drive upon which all past, present, and even potential future events are recorded. In other words, the DNA informs our personal physical reality, and the *Akashic Record,* cosmic in proportion, records and informs our soul's journey.

Just as thought is impressed on the clear field of mind, so are one's deeds and actions recorded in the Akashic Record, variously called the Book of Life or the Hall of Records. On the temple walls in Egypt one often sees the ibis-headed man form of Thoth, scribe of the gods, with stylus in hand, recording the offerings or deeds of Pharaoh into the book of his soul's record of millions of years. There are various other depictions of Seshet recording specific deeds of Pharaoh in the *Renpit,* the leaves of life, which are the records of the years on the tree of life. She notches a palm frond, tracking personal lives, while Thoth records the cosmic history. According to my friend Normandi Ellis (scholar and author on the Egyptian Mysteries), Thoth is the overseer and Seshet is the record keeper. Although this was not called the Akashic Record by ancient Egyptians, I believe that this is the current name for that ancient process, and it relates as well to the concept resurrected by Madam Blavatsky and the Western magical tradition.

The records hold the information contained in the blueprint formed within Akasha. On a personal level, they indicate the direction of our individual lives and what brought us to where we are in any given moment. The potential future emanates from where we are at the present and includes every possible outcome.

This blueprint of the collective holds the entire history of what has ever been, what is, and what may be. At any given moment, it is possible to retrieve that information if one has access to the Akashic realm.

It is one thing to witness changes or to let things take their natural course, and it is another to have a hand in healing through conscious participation while working with Akasha.

The easiest way to comprehend the Akashic Record is through direct experience, as it is hard to articulate in words. In my book, *Power Animal Meditations,* there is a chapter that not only describes but also takes you through an experience of the Akashic Record through guided visualization. I recommend that you try it.

AKASHIC PRACTICES

Akasha is the most important element in Alchemical Healing; however, by itself, it will not provide the intended results. Akasha must be used in relation to the other four elements, which must be in perfect harmony and balance. Once the practitioner feels and can sustain that resonance, she can move outside of time and space as we know it and accomplish work that cannot be concluded in our three-dimensional reality. Perhaps this is the *dreamtime* of the Australian Aboriginals. By whatever name you call it, the realm of Akasha is certainly a dimension where shamans go—accomplishing what seem like impossible feats of fasting and journeying—to retrieve information, power, and healing for their communities.

★ ☽ ★

Use the following technique to refresh the Akasha for yourself or for another person. Start with practicing on yourself. As always your intention is most important; you must work from your heart and hold feelings of well-being and compassion. You are connecting directly with the intelligence and consciousness of each cell as well as with Akasha, while asking for a clear and perfect blueprint for yourself, so that you will be able to function in good health on physical, emotional, mental, and spiritual levels.

Remember, you may experience a drowsy, almost drugged state when working with Akasha. It is through repeated practice and determination that you can develop the ability to maintain full consciousness.

EXERCISE

Refreshing the Akasha

Start by grounding and centering, using your word, and bringing up your caduceus, devoting extra attention at the heart chakra to become clear and centered.

Set your intention on refreshing the Akashic blueprint. See yourself sitting within a glowing egg. Reach up and draw the symbol for Akasha, using the Akashic fingers (the middle ones). Akasha begins to flow from the opening, slowly dribbling, filling the egg to overflowing with rich, purple-black honey and drizzling down the sides. The entire auric egg is being filled from the top so that the inside and outside take on the deep purple color of Akasha.

Hold to feelings of compassion and well-being. This process is pushing out the old Akasha from the inside, completely replacing it while you are holding your attention on renewing your clear and perfect Akashic blueprint.

As the egg becomes full, a pattern forms inside the purple color. This pattern permeates deep within the egg. It can appear as energy, pictures, a multidimensional web, or whatever unique perception comes to you. It may be through energetic awareness and feeling, rather than your sense of sight, that you come to recognize this three-dimensional grid. It forms according to the intent and the need of the individual while you feed it the love and life energy from your hands. You will know that the crystallization of the pattern is complete because there are no further developments or changes in the pattern and there is a sensation that you are no longer generating energy from your heart or hands. Simply disconnect when the process is complete, and ground yourself. Sometimes it helps to touch the ground.

Make note of how this practice feels the first time you use it, and again how it strengthens when you repeat it. If you are part of a study group, you might try this as a group exercise. When working in a group, you can all draw Akasha into the same egg. As a collective effort you can enlarge the size of the egg—and you will notice a greater flow of Akasha and perhaps an infusion of information on a more collective level.

Every time you refresh your Akasha, you're allowing subtle shifts that will be reflected in the future. You as a sentient individual, and you as a representative of the collective consciousness, are co-creating with the matrix of creation when you do this exercise.

USING AKASHA FOR HEALING

Both physical and psychological problems yield to healing that utilizes Akasha. You can use it within a healing to reach a deeper level of communication with the various parts of the body or psyche. When working with psychological problems and systemic diseases, send the energies to the entire body rather than to a specific organ, tumor, injury, or illness. This process brings healing to the entire auric system. When you enter Akasha for information on psychological issues, you may uncover layers of personal, family, group, or planetary history. Wherever the problem resides, its residence becomes evident to either the person receiving the healing, or the practitioner. As the practitioner, I suggest you first attempt to have the person find that information for herself, before you offer any insights from your own perception.

Alchemical Healing can be similar to baking: you put all the ingredients together and fire it up with energy. When you use Akasha, however, it is especially important to avoid imposing your personal will into the design that you are manifesting. With Akasha, it is vital to allow the unseen mystery to guide your way. You have plenty of skill to bring to the work—your ability to manifest the elements, invoke the totems and other allies, utilize smudge and other techniques of purification for yourself and your client, and direct the energies. You must be willing to ask for the help you need.

Because it is informative, Akasha is a necessary ingredient for learning about anything. If you wished to know what it would feel like to be a part of something, or to have some specific kind of knowledge, you could gather up the Akasha within yourself and project yourself into whatever it is you wish to know about. As you gain mastery, you can merge with the intended source of knowledge to move into specific situations or experiences.

You can use the following healing form on its own or within a healing that you have already started or whenever you sense the need for repatterning the DNA. This might include healing old injuries, genetic diseases, or emotional or mental habit patterns that are especially difficult to dislodge. Use it also in those healings that your intuition tells you are appropriate. Please note that this form utilizes the four principles of Alchemical Healing as stated in Chapter 19.

EXERCISE
Akashic Healing Technique

Akasha carries levels of information that have to do with group consciousness and group history, including collective trauma, plus information about ancestral lines. Using Akasha in the following way, you can help heal patterns resulting from deep trauma and old schisms, injury, or disease.

Remember to maintain your clarity and focus. If you work from an unbalanced frame of mind, you can distort the pattern and, although you may not harm the person you are working on, you run the risk of getting yourself stuck in a maze of confusion. It is better to halt the process and go about it with a different set of techniques than to continue and risk confusion or distortion.

Start by drawing the Akashic symbol, using your Akasha fingers, and pulling Akasha into the work through the portal you have just created. Direct the Akasha toward the area with which you are working. You can feel it, almost like thick deep purple space.

As you pour Akasha into the person, he or she might have the sensation of being surrounded by an inky purple-black velvet blanket. After a moment, when the Akasha has permeated the place where you've directed it, focus your intention and attention. When you become clear you will be able to perceive the inception of whatever problem you're working on—and its future probabilities, as well. As healer, you can observe (and can direct the person you're working with to observe), with compassion and non-judgment, the information that begins to reveal itself. It may come as a feeling, a picture, as short as a flash or as long as a movie. It may deal with things as small as a family issue or as large as matters of global significance.

It helps if both healer and patient drop their investment in the outcome. Expectations stifle the process. Simply observe, acknowledge, and accept the information without judgment. Once honored, the disruptive pattern that underlies the problem is absorbed into Akasha, or allowed to pass through the Akasha, which works like a universal solvent to dissolve and release its imprint. Whenever you and the person you are working with feel the resulting harmony, wash away the old habit or illness with the element Water, which will clear up any residual toxicity. You may wish to use pure, clear elemental Water, and/or augment its power with an appropriate medicinal plant spirit. Grounding the healing in Earth helps to set the new pattern as well as bring you back into a functioning state of consciousness in this plane. Allies may be invited in at any time to help during this process.

It will be obvious to you when the transformation is complete. If a symbol was observed when Akasha was first invoked, it will have transformed to one of a more positive nature. If a story was revealed, it would have been resolved. Symptoms may have abated, or in some way shifted. There will be an intuitive recognition of completion.

Be sure to offer your love, life energy, and gratitude. Once the process is complete and you have broken your connection, the doorway that you used no longer exists.

It is usually best if the client accesses the information directly, rather than being led by the healer. Sometimes the person cannot perceive on his own. Akasha, by its nature, is often difficult to comprehend for someone who lacks experience. In that case, you can give some guidance according to your own interpretation but check with the person to see if he resonates with whatever you are relaying. Pay close attention. If you are incorrect in your interpretation, it will not resonate with the client. Always remember that the person with whom you are working is very open during this process. It is vital to allow him as much opportunity as possible to find the root causes and underlying patterns for himself.

Traumatic events do not need to be relived in order for this technique to be effective. The healer's job is to hold space and pour in Akasha and other elements as appropriate to further the alchemical process of transformation. When the symbol is transformed, there will be change regardless of what is revealed—an individual incident, distorted family trauma, collective violence, or global catastrophe. When the issue is dissolved in Akasha it no longer has the same impact on the current physical or emotional reality.

While you have been holding space during the alchemical transmutation, the old pattern has been displaced by a new and healthy pattern. In a physical healing, every cell is forming according to the new blueprint and is taking the place of the ones that you are allowing to dissolve. In an emotional healing, the habit patterns are being rearranged so that the basis of response is altered.

Increased complexity and difficulty requires a more varied bag of tools and skill.

When you are working with Akasha, remember that you are holding space for something *other* to happen, and for a new level of intuitive engagement. Your skill lies in maintaining clear intention, focus, and balance for as long as it takes. Any sounds that are happening around you, or whatever might be seen as a distraction within the realm of your sensitivities, is grist for the mill and can be incorporated into the healing. If random thoughts appear or you begin to get confused, it is time to call for help from the myriad allies supporting this work. With absolute focused attention, you will know which of your tools to apply along the way.

STORIES OF AKASHIC HEALINGS

The following story came from a class taught by Bo Clark in Cloudland, Georgia. In it, one of her students, Allison, relates what happened to her during a practice session with another student, Lisa.

> As I lay on the table, I focused on relaxing. My knee was whining for attention in the way it has for a very long time.
>
> Over the years, I'd gone to different doctors complaining about my knee. Handing over a fistful of drugs and giving a pat on the back, they told me, "That's as good as it gets, and at your age, you will be experiencing those little aches and pains," or "If the pills don't work, we will consider surgery." In class, Lisa chose to work with me. It became a group healing with her directing. Bo was close by to observe. The knee was hurting and was very "hot."
>
> First she called on the element Water, hoping to put out the fire, to cool the knee down. I felt my leg swelling and getting tight. In fact, it became very uncomfortable. Dagny put an etheric drain in my foot. That relieved the pressure but the knee was still hot. It was still hurting. Lisa was not comfortable with asking for Akasha, but she knew the knee was holding this pain.

She called on Akasha, and I felt myself going back, way back to when I was a little girl. To a time before the knee knew pain.

It was summertime and the carnival had come to our town. There was cotton candy, clowns, a Ferris wheel, and other kiddie rides. The only things I cared about were the ponies. All I wanted to do was ride the ponies. It's hard being a city dweller when the heart is filled with country. My folks are city through and through. While they were watching my baby brother ride the little cars, I noticed one of the ponies all alone munching hay. The little fellow was just on the other side of the rope. I was short enough to walk right under the rope. The pony raised his head while still munching a mouthful of hay and invited me over. He stretched his head forward to inspect me. My heart went racing with this close connection. The pony's eyes were soft and wise.

Suddenly, I was knocked to the ground. My knee hit metal. I was shocked, angry, confused, and embarrassed. Owweywwow, my knee really hurt. I looked up to see my father. He had knocked me down, away from the pony, because he was afraid it would hurt me, and he was upset. He scooped me up and proceeded to admonish me for my errant behavior. I tried to tell him I only wanted to say "hi" and pet the pony. I tried to tell him that the pony would not hurt me. I was given all the reasons why what I wanted was not safe or good. It didn't matter what he said. I was hurt, emotionally and physically. My knee was cut and bleeding. My heart was broken. Dad knew how much I loved horses. And I was his little girl. Why wouldn't he believe me?

Was this the moment I replaced animal communication with fear?

Back in the class, I was aware that someone close and familiar was asking me questions and guiding me through this past memory. I was asked if I could forgive my father. It took some time to process this question. When I said "Yes," it was as though a dam burst. My heart, body, and soul flooded with emotion—the emotion of unconditional love. My father was forgiven on many levels that day. Still working with Akasha, the dark angry memory was replaced with one more plausible and filled with light and love.

With this shift, a peace spread over me. I found myself floating in a sunlit stream, waving like a strand of sea grass. Water tumbled over me, rocking me gently in its moving wake, yet I felt anchored soundly in the rocks. The element of Earth was used to support the healing of the knee. It felt rather like cold wet sand packed firmly around the knee. The bubbling, cleansing water continued to flow, carrying the emotional slime to the big waters where it would be dispersed.

I was cold when I returned to the present. Grounded and grateful, we ended the session. My knee was no longer carrying the cold, yet fiery, pain.

This next story of another healing done by Kathryn Ravenwood demonstrates the creativity that can be brought into healings using Akasha. Remember, Alchemical Healing is an art form, and once you are comfortable with the palette, you can begin to play more freely.

V. was excited about starting to ride horseback again, but soon after she started she had a bad fall and hurt her hip. Now she was afraid to get back on the horse. She asked me to help ease the pain in her hip and get her through the fear so that she could ride again. She asked specifically for the Alchemical Healing work, as we had worked that way on other issues.

I started by drawing Akasha and bringing it in around her. As soon as I felt the Akasha moving in, I asked her to go back to a time before the accident, a time when she was riding a horse and feeling really happy about it.

I could tell she was there because she smiled, which was my cue to withdraw a thread of purple aka out of the place where she had this joyful feeling. I pulled it out of her smile and her heart and grounded it through her body and into the earth. This was done step by step out loud, with V. fully participating. Then I asked her to remember earlier in the day she fell and what it felt like as she was on her way to ride the horse. I called on more Akasha. When V. got that happy feeling of looking forward to the ride, I again went in and took threads of aka and pulled them out through her belly and her sacrum, and anchored them down into the ground once more. Next I wanted her to let me know what it felt like to be up riding the horse before the fall. This was also joyful, and again I anchored that feeling with threads of aka into the earth.

Finally I took her to the time when she had the fall. I reminded her that we could not change that the fall happened, but could perhaps change how she landed and how she felt about it. V. said okay, and as she remembered falling, I had her go in slow motion. A big net came under her and broke her fall and then lowered her down onto a huge, soft mattress on the ground. When she hit the ground the shock was lessened, as though she were landing on a fluffy pillow.

Now I pulled up all the anchors, all the aka cords, brought them up through her sacrum and her belly, and braided them together into purple-and-gold-flecked reins that I threaded through the horse's bridle, and from there into V.'s hands. I suggested she get back on Skippy and continue her ride.

As we completed the session, V. thanked the horse and made sure he was well taken care of before she returned to the room where we were working.

After this one session, her fear and her pain were completely gone, and she felt excited at the prospect of riding again. She feels that this experience will help her become a better rider, because she will feel more connected to her mount.

ADVANCED AKASHA EMPOWERMENT

After you have worked for some time with Akasha and have developed a level of comfort with using this element, it will be time to receive the next Akashic empowerment. This comes in the form of a meditation that is also a practice that should be done periodically.

This practice is useful for grounding yourself in Akasha, balancing yourself, and connecting with the overseeing council that will become more familiar as you return again and again. The first time you enter into this practice is most certainly an initiation.

(It is recommended that you receive the Caduceus Empowerment before you enter into this meditation.)

INITIATION

STAR COUNCIL MEDITATION

Be very comfortable, sitting on floor or chair, with your back as straight as possible. Breathe deeply and allow yourself to become fully relaxed. It is quite useful to bring up your caduceus so that you are centered and balanced, with a strong current of energy moving through your body. . . . Feel the energy running through you, showering you until you feel very clean, clear, and centered within your High Self. It is very important to be heart centered before continuing.

Imagine a pyramid with four sides in the proportions of the Great Pyramid at Giza, and perceive it coming up from beneath you, slightly bigger than your body. The pyramid is made of solid Akasha, pure Akasha, deep purple-black in color. It comes up from underneath and rises so that the tip is above you and the foundation is below, and you are in the middle, completely surrounded inside this pyramid of Akasha. . . .

A second pyramid of Akasha pointing downward from above drops down and intersects with the one you are in. When it comes to rest, you are sitting in the middle of a perfect, three-dimensional, ten-pointed star, with your heart at the center. The facets that you see from the inside make it look like a deep indigo diamond-cut gemstone. . . .

When the two pyramids are in place and you are centered in the middle of the diamond, it begins to glow, inside and outside. . . . The purple indigo color lightens and brightens until you are in a clear diamond with many facets, and the diamond starts to spin to your left. You stay stationary and the diamond spins around you. There is light inside and outside, and the diamond starts slow and picks up speed as it spins, faster and faster and faster. The light is refracting through all the facets. . . .

While this is spinning to the left (important) there is another set of indigo pyramids of Akasha coming up from the bottom and down from the top. They are just a little bigger than the first ones. They come into place, the same as the first ones did, and you are again in the center, the midpoint. You can perceive this second indigo diamond just a little way out from the one that you are in as it spins. . . . This second diamond also begins to glow and clarify. It grows clear and bright and slowly begins to turn to the right, then speeds up. The first is still going to the left. The new one picks up speed until it is going equally fast to the right. . . .

Notice the feeling in your heart. Notice any fluctuations in your life energy. There is an intense light display from all the spinning facets. As they spin, your electromagnetic field increases. Your level of consciousness skyrockets. While maintaining presence in this meditation, you are rebuilding circuitry, balancing, cleaning, stabilizing, and preparing for the future. . . .

All around you the reflections of the light are dazzling. After some time, this attracts the attention of the Star Council of which Thoth is a part. They will come and observe, direct, counsel, and adjust or do healing on you. Hold your focus while maintaining awareness of the council and allowing any interaction that might be available. . . .

When your time with the council is complete, while still deep into the feelings generated by the experience of being within the spinning pyramids, open your eyes. This allows you to begin to bring this practice into ordinary reality as well as into the realm of deep meditation.

Hold still in this place for as long as you can—a minimum of ten minutes when you first start. During subsequent practice you will gradually be able to hold it longer and longer and longer. If you are able to concentrate longer than ten minutes the first time, keep present with it until you start to fade and become distracted. . . .

After you have completed the practice and grounded in your ordinary reality, it would be of benefit to practice yoga, dance, or go for a walk to help bring this powerful work into your body in a physical way.

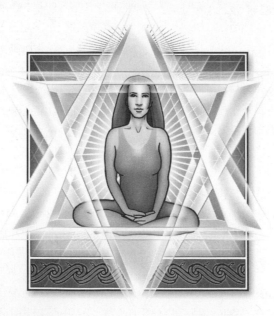

Figure 15.1. Star Council Meditation

16
ADVANCED HEALING TECHNIQUES

DIRECT CONDUCTING OF ENERGIES

When the energies were first introduced and accessed, you were taught to gather the energy that needed to be removed from the body and to conduct it into the earth, water, or wherever appropriate, with a prayer for its transformation into its highest potential. As you become more accustomed to this manner of working, it becomes a fluid movement and you find a variety of ways to conduct the energy from one place to another.

After you have received and practiced the Caduceus Empowerment and have developed enough confidence in the work to be totally at ease, you may begin to conduct these undesirable energies directly into the earth or wherever you have chosen. To perform the transfer most efficiently, simply direct your generative hand (usually the right) or fingertips toward the appropriate receptacle, usually the earth, at the same time you are pulling or holding the place for release with your other hand (usually the left). When you work in this way, the energy appears to move through you instantly; yet there is no danger of it getting caught in your body. It is as though it makes an electrical arc from one point of contact to the other. If, however, you have any doubts or feel uncomfortable conducting virulent energies through your body, then stick with the original technique as taught in Chapter 12 for removing energies.

To make this technique for removing energies more elegant, envision a clear channel, like a meridian, moving from your receiving hand up your arm and across your shoulders, then down the other side and into the earth or receptacle of water, out to the sun, or to wherever you are intending it to go for safekeeping and transformation.

ADVANCED ALCHEMICAL FORMULA

There is no end to the rudiments or elements that are available for inclusion in Alchemical Healing. Tools from all paths and traditions contribute elements that are useful. The criteria for selecting tools happens "in the moment," and no set recipe will work the same way every time for any specific illness, although there certainly are propensities.

As the body of work that appears in these pages developed, the tools unique to Thoth's direct influence were recorded and practiced in conjunction with traditional Western medical therapies and adjunctive alternative therapies, in an inclusive way. In the course of the research, certain patterns emerged that work effectively with speed and elegance, and I pass these on to you here; however, it is important not to be fettered by rules or structures that become arbitrary and thus destroy the spirit of the art. These techniques combine to create a healing art form whose very life depends upon spontaneity. It is magic that, if overly formulated or stripped of its mystery, becomes stagnant and ineffectual.

Most of the tools can be used independently, and each should be practiced for some time before trying to put it all together in the following sequence, which is the closest to a formula this work offers. Once you have had significant experience with the element Akasha, and have gained comfort using all the techniques previously described, you will be able to do this with ease.

Advanced Healing Practice

This alchemical process requires containment, a kind of hermetically sealed alchemical vessel. When working this alchemy on someone—either on the entire body, on an organ, or even on emotional problems—we first use Earth to build the container, which works like an oven or a crucible, within which the process of transmutation occurs. Begin as you would any healing, preparing yourself by raising the caduceus, setting your intention, and using your word.

Draw a cube, the three-dimensional symbol of Earth, in the air with your Earth fingers, indicating what you want to enclose, and invoke the energy of Earth to build the container. The cubic structure of the element Earth gives stability to the container and helps to hold the body safe during the process of transformation. Within this hermetically sealed vessel you can direct the appropriate elements to produce the desired changes.

Akasha is the first element you infuse into the situation. Draw the symbol of Akasha and focus your attention and intention on filling the vessel with the inky violet-black medium. Your intention is to retrieve the information that Akasha holds, the blueprint or patterning of the problem, at its source.

It is usually helpful to engage the person you are working with. Even if you are a seer and can retrieve the information directly, it is more beneficial for the person to find the information for herself, with whatever symbols, images, or insights are presented. Usually once the person is enveloped in the Akasha (which can feel like a blue-black mist or an inky black velvet blanket), an image, recollection, or sense of the source of the problem will emerge out of the darkness. Often it is perceived as a memory. It might play out as a movie or fly by as a fleeting image. It might be a static symbol, usually with some darkness or negative connotation, such as a black cross, a barbed wire fence, or a dead tree. Suggest that your client apply all her senses to the retrieval of this information.

When a symbol or story becomes apparent, you can begin to use the other elements to continue the transformation process.

Usually I use Fire at this stage because I wish to break down the old pattern as it is no longer useful. Fire can be followed by Air to fuel the fire and combust the energies represented by the symbolism. When I want to heat up the fire I go back and forth between Fire and Air while intending Fire. In some situations if Fire feels too harsh, use Water in its place. Whatever you use to transform the energies, follow with Akasha in order to absorb any waste products generated from the combustion, regardless of whether it is through calcination, dissolution, or both. With this process no conduction into the earth is necessary because the energies get absorbed directly by the Akasha, returning back to their source, as the whole work continues to be contained within the earthen vessel. It is like a dance with the elements, a play that moves from one element to the next with grace. There is no need to close out of one to go into another. Encourage the person being treated to give feedback throughout the process, so you may respond appropriately at any given moment.

Music can be a key element in this form, although it is not required. I have worked with many different styles of music, usually chosen to suit the individual and the problem—anything from drums to classical to Gregorian chants to Grateful Dead. The remarkable thing is that whatever the music, if carefully selected, it seems to work with the healing as though it is alive, and the instrumentation reflects the elements used at the exact moment. The music seems to penetrate the process, adding a dimension where light and sound intersect with matter, and so the effect is intensified.

As you work the elements with the intention of dissolving the basic patterning of the problem, whether physical or emotional, there will be indications that report the progress. The images, symbols, or feelings change from negative to neutral, and then they transform into new, more positive images that indicate that the healing is taking place. Be sure to allow time for the changes to occur.

At any time during this process, you can introduce animal and herbal allies and consult spirit guides to bring other elements into the mix. Each moment seems to direct the next activity, and you are always guided by a balanced combination of intuition and practicality.

When a new scenario or symbol, healthy and colorful, is fully formed, it is time to seal the newly created pattern of health. You can run some of the element of Water for a final rinse before setting the new pattern in Earth. Use the element Earth at the end to ground and stabilize the work. Earth also helps bring this subtle, more spiritual work into our three-dimensional, physical world. When the healing feels complete, thank all of the beings that helped you, then break the connection. It is always a wonder when the music (if you've chosen to use it) functions in synch with the work, and closure is natural and complete. The Earth oven or alchemical vessel will dissolve once it is no longer needed.

PSYCHIC SURGERY

I first encountered the term *psychic surgery* during my first class with Nadia. There was a dentist in the circle who, when asked his intention for being in the class, replied that he wanted to learn psychic surgery. Nadia was almost off-hand in her response when she said that, of course, it would be taught in her workshop.

The idea of psychic surgery fascinated me, but it was difficult to find much written about it back in 1982. I found an article that described several South American psychic surgeons, one of whom was reported to be working with several dead Western physicians who were guiding his hands. According to the article, he would speak the language of whichever doctor he was working with in the moment, and he could enter the body and remove all manner of ailments without leaving any scars.

I was intrigued. I decided that I wanted to learn to heal in that way, so I conducted a ceremony during which I offered to serve in a similar way, and asked Creator of the Mystery to send me a doctor from the spirit world to assist with my work. I then continued on about my studies and consequent teaching. It was a number of years later that I looked around during a healing and to my surprise realized that my prayer had been answered. Indeed I did and still do have a team of surgeons, and we most certainly work together. There are Bear and Cobra, Thoth and the Crone, a Tibetan magician, Sekhmet, and Kuan Yin, to name just a few.

A better term for this form of psychic surgery might be *etheric surgery*, because that term would not carry the identification with the Philippine and Brazilian forms, which are actually somewhat different. Philippine healers often employ dramatic tactics for effect while practicing a variety of excellent healing skills. Sometimes there is a fine line between sham and shamanism.

It is human nature to believe what we see and feel. If our subconscious mind has reason to believe something is true, it doesn't necessarily distinguish between our three-dimensional, consensus-based reality and other realms or dimensions. If you have a lucid dream, your body will respond as though what happened in that dream is a fact of life. Your subconscious mind responds to events that occur on any level of reality as if they were true. Therefore, if you have an experience that is seen or heard or felt during which healing occurs, it is likely that, even if the event happened in trance or in another dimension, there will be a physical result. If a person feels your hands inside his body and feels the change in the depth of pain, that result will often continue in his everyday physical reality.

EXERCISE

Practicing Psychic Surgery Techniques

To begin a psychic surgery it is important to be grounded and centered, so be sure to have your caduceus and your allies in place. Start the procedure as you would any other healing, connecting with the Universal Life Force energy and scanning the individual to make the strongest connection and to get as much information as possible. Remove all undesirable energies that can be released easily, and determine exactly where you want to make the incision. The idea is to create an opening through which you can reach a deeper level, perhaps the subatomic, microcosmic arena in which it is easier to manipulate the molecules within the dense tissue.

Turn on the energy and make sure you have a strong connection as you sweep the area like a metal detector. You are not touching the body, but your hands, with your fingers together, are about six inches more or less above the skin or clothing. Mark likes to make his connection from about two inches off of the body; then, once the connection is made, he moves out to about four to six inches. Neither clothing, bandages, nor casts will get in the way. Turn your right hand (left, if left-handed) so that your fingertips are pointing toward the area you have selected. With your intention, condense the light that radiates from your fingertips into a fine beam like a laser. Again, it will become concentrated in accordance with your intention. Use your power word as a booster. The incision is made by using the light like a laser beam. Make the cut only as large as you need to accomplish the work at hand. You might bring your hands closer to the body while you are actually drawing the condensed beam the length of the opening you wish to make. To the person this might feel like a needle being drawn across the skin.

When you've made the incision, you must open it by placing your hands over the cut, palm facing palm. Then, with tremendous focus and intention, pull your hands slowly apart from one another, and you will feel resistance as the opening is created. Again, this is a good time to add the power of your word. Check with the person to see what he or she is feeling. Most people feel as though the area has actually opened. This has been described as a feeling of vulnerability or, simply, being open.

Once the person has been opened, immediately change the intention for the energy to a soft light, with the accompanying message to the internal tissues that the visit is friendly. You have entered a subatomic realm where everything is of the microcosm and is exposed, and it is important to be even more sensitive and careful than usual. The work continues in the same manner as any other healing; however, there is a palpable sense of being inside the body of the person you are working on. When you check in with the person now, you may find that he feels as though your hands are on his physical body, or even inside it.

You can continue with removing, building, nurturing with herbs, or whatever techniques are required in the moment. It is important to hold your focus and concentration on the work at hand, and hold space vigilantly throughout this process. Regardless of which aspects of Alchemical Healing you apply, it is imperative to lavish the person with light and life force energy before completing the surgery. When you have sensed that the work is done, it is vital that you close the incision, at every level of the auric field. To do this, bring your hands back together, palm to palm, with intention and focus over the opening, as you feel the coming together of the tissue and skin. Start with the incision at the level of the skin, then smooth over the place with your hands several inches out from the body. Continue smoothing at ever higher levels above the body until you are sure there are no more open places—no tears in the field where energy can leak out—and the auric field has been returned to full integrity. Then take a moment to disconnect and thank the spirits and allies who helped you with the work.

If the person can describe the details of what a medical surgeon would do, you can often translate those methods into the realm of Alchemical Healing. I have had several successful psychic surgeries working on and with doctors who have guided me through the process. I can substitute etheric drains in order to siphon off swelling, use an etheric comfrey paste as glue, and be as creative as my imagination will allow in order to accomplish the necessary changes using practical means. It's a great opportunity to apply one's practical intellect with one's intuition and imagination.

PSYCHIC SURGERY STORIES

Here is an example from an Alchemical Healing class taught by Bo Clark in Cloudland, Georgia. Bo reports as follows:

I was excited about the upcoming Alchemical Healing class, as something inside told me this was going to be an extremely powerful one. The class went well and there were many new awakenings throughout the weekend. One of the women had brought her nineteen-year-old daughter, Bree. They had been here several times before but Bree had never studied healing.

Toward the end of the workshop we ventured into psychic surgery. I did a brief demonstration on a woman with a jaw problem. I then had the class break into groups of two to practice, suggesting that they use any of the elements or techniques they had learned during the weekend. Bree immediately asked the woman she was to work with to lie on her stomach. She placed her hands on the woman's right shoulder area and surrounded the area with golden light that flowed from her newly opened hands and fingertips.

She began to organize her tools for psychic surgery. I was surprised to see her go that way, as she had no previous experience in this arena, and I was drawn to focus on her procedure. Bree followed her instincts and trusted without question! She gathered her tools from the ethers, sterilized them, and made an incision in the woman's shoulder. Carefully and methodically she went through all the layers with such precision that one could almost see the tools and the surgery. We certainly could feel their energy. After making the incision she began to make a rubbing motion. I asked what she was doing, and she told me that something was there that needed to be removed or filed down. She continued this for about twenty minutes. Bree's intention was clear and her ability to focus was quite amazing. She then said that she felt it was gone, cleaned it with the Water element, packed Earth around it, and began, once again methodically, to close up the incision.

The woman who had received this surgery had a big grin on her face when she was done. She then shared that X rays had been taken earlier that week that showed she had a bone spur in her shoulder. The doctor told her she might need it removed, as it was very painful and also interfered with her range of movement. Bree asked her how she felt now, and the woman smiled and said the pain was gone and she had more mobility. She said, "I am going to go back and have another X ray taken this week." She reported back later that same week that the bone spur was in fact gone. Needless to say, the doctor was amazed.

★ ☽ ★

The form of psychic surgery I was originally taught and have since developed is bloodless. When I first discovered how effective this method of healing was, I did it often, with little restraint. Although I still find it to be a powerful tool, I have since learned discernment. Occasionally people have a reaction to psychic surgery the same as if they had been through a medical, under-the-knife surgery. When that happens, they must treat themselves to recuperation time; sometimes they require bed rest for a few days. More rarely I have had people go into shock and require further special attention. In such situations, all other obligations fade, and I stay with them until they stabilize.

Only work with this method if you are willing and prepared to see it through, and you know that the person has time to recover and honor the process. And it is especially important to be sure the person is either sitting or lying down, and has been advised about the possibility of requiring recuperation time.

As a result of the following story and a few similar experiences, psychic surgery has become a method of last resort that I use only when a person is too armored to reach by a less invasive technique, or when I am specifically guided to do so.

★ ☽ ★

The son of an old friend of mine, Peter, was badly injured when he fell about twenty feet off of a deck and landed in a cement courtyard. He left his body and was looking down from above when he heard the sirens and saw the fire truck and ambulance arriving. He immediately slammed back into his body and got up and ran away. When he returned home he tried to tell the people with whom he lived that he was hurt, but they were young and self-consumed, and he wasn't bleeding, so they didn't heed his requests for help.

I happened to drop by about ten days later to visit someone who lived in the same house. Peter was there and still in considerable pain. He told me what had happened, and I offered to try to help.

As I tried to feel and see what was wrong, I couldn't get past the armor he had built to keep the pain at bay.

I asked him for permission to go deeper into his body. He was still standing up when I made the incision. Big mistake! I had to move quickly to catch him as he fell. Within about ten seconds his color turned totally ashen, he broke out in a cold and clammy sweat, and he started to convulse. Through my surprise I took a deep breath, centered myself, and asked for help. What came to me was that since he did not die when he fell, he would not die now. Rather, he was experiencing the shock that he had initially cast aside in order to make his escape. To compensate, he had gone rigid and had been holding it all together by sheer force of will since the accident happened. When I made the incision my penetration unraveled his defenses, and the house of cards came tumbling down. Now, what was protected lay bare. I placed my left hand flat a few inches above his back and began slowly and gently circling counterclockwise, firmly yet sensitively pulling, like a magnet or vacuum cleaner as described earlier. I could feel his body release the trauma and pain; it felt like drawing raw scrambled eggs through a straw. The distressed energy accumulated in my hand and I offered it to the earth before returning for a second gather. I then refilled the entire region of his body with love and light and healing herbs, and carefully closed the field where I had made the incision.

As a result of our work, he was able to relax and begin the actual healing process, and to find considerable relief from the pain of his injuries.

★ ☽ ★

I have had uncanny success working with various knee injuries and problems. Many have required psychic surgery, such as the following example:

Some years ago I had an opportunity to work with an emergency room physician who was considering knee surgery. Because of his professional knowledge and expertise, he was able to describe to me exactly what needed to be accomplished and how the surgeon would go about it if he were to choose conventional surgery. In essence, he guided me through the procedure, which I was able to translate into my own psychic surgical techniques. He was very sensitive and could not only feel everything that was happening, he could articulate, so that we knew we were sharing the same experience from our distinct perspectives. I remember the look on his face when, at the end of the session, he moved his knee back and forth, stood up to test his weight upon it, and declared himself completely healed. We then went for a walk to the top of a nearby hill that would have been out of the question before the psychic surgery. That was many, many years ago, and to my knowledge the symptoms have not returned.

This is from Danielle Hoffman:

> Right after I took a course in Alchemical Healing, which included psychic surgery, I was at the beach with my adopted parents. My dad (a bit of a skeptic) had a bone spur on his heel which was preventing him from truly enjoying his vacation because it made walking his dogs on the beach uncomfortable. So I offered to do some healing with him and he agreed.
>
> First I pulled away all of the material that was ready to come out and put it into the earth. It was then that I realized the source of his problem was much deeper than I was reaching. We talked about the psychic surgery I was learning and I warned him that he would need to rest after the procedure. He agreed to let me try it.
>
> After calling in all my guides I extended the light out of the tips of my right hand in a laser and made an incision. Once opened, I began to carve away gently at the additional pieces of bone that were causing problems. I asked him to focus on releasing what he no longer needed and to think about his favorite animal and color.
>
> After removing the spur, I showered the area with Water mixed with herbs that I was given by Grandmother Bear. Then

I poured more energy in to fill the cavity back up and carefully closed the opening I had made. My dad and I talked a little bit more about his interpretations of the deeper indications that the bone spur represented for him, and we were able to release thought forms that were the root cause of the problem, with assistance from Sekhmet and the element Akasha.

Over the next few days, my dad experienced relief similar to the relief he had gotten through massage in the past. When we next talked about it a few months later, he told me the bone spur had completely vanished and that he had no more pain. It is now three years later and he still has not had any recurrence of the symptoms or the spur.

Also from Danielle:

I was teaching my first Alchemical Healing, Level II class and planned to do a psychic surgery demonstration during the weekend. I had only used this technique a handful of times over the years, simply because I can usually accomplish whatever I need with the assistance of my guides and the support I receive. This generally makes an opening unnecessary.

I wanted the perfect demonstration and was eyeing everyone in the class for the entire weekend to see who it might be. One woman had really severe endometriosis, which is also what I have been dealing with, so I wondered if I would be able to stay detached and clear working with her. I asked Thoth who would be the best person to work with and of course it was she.

We prepared to do this psychic surgery as a group. Before we began I asked for and got a thorough history of her endometriosis and some key things about her life. The symptoms of her endometriosis included a combination of intense pain and swelling, and a constant emotional roller coaster ride.

We started the healing by clearing the area and making a

strong connection. I then went in through Akasha and made the incision from there.

Once the incision had been made and we entered, it was incredibly hot inside. Some of her personal guides came, one of whom was the Crone, who gave her some flowers and herbs, including lavender.

We then began to work on clearing past abuse issues that Akasha revealed by traveling into and through that time of her life and into her ancestral lineage. We asked the guides to find the original blueprint before the abuse occurred. While they were finding it, we began to clear away the chocolate-like adhesions that were all around her ovaries, fallopian tubes, and even her bladder. We cauterized the adhesions with the help of Fire and Air to help burn them away, then followed with a wash of herbs and Water.

The woman herself actively participated in the releasing and clearing. When the guides gifted us with the original blueprint, Spider showed up to weave it into place. We then created a lavender mist over her entire body to relax and harmonize the emotions. All of us filled the area with light and love and envisioned it whole and complete.

After offering a great amount of gratitude to the guides, we closed the incision and applied an herbal salve to the wound. We then closed and sealed her aura and released the work. I thanked all that participated.

It was several months before I had occasion to see this woman again. She told me that after that day she no longer had any symptoms related to the endometriosis.

★ ☽ ★

There are times when the same level of work can be accomplished without making an incision if you have a highly developed perception of the energy. Occasionally folks are brought to my Alchemical Healing classes because their needs are perfect for demonstration. There was a forty-year-old woman, pregnant with her first child. She was seven months along and was facing her remaining time bed-ridden because of danger posed from the intrusion of a huge fibroid tumor, inoperable under the circumstances. She was otherwise quite healthy, very athletic and strong. The fibroid was vying with the fetus for space, and it was a tricky situation that necessitated bed rest and a cesarean to deliver the baby when it came to term.

I began the work as usual; however, I extended my energies carefully into the woman's uterus and established communication with the fetus before doing anything else. I got an immediate sense of knowing that psychic surgery was not appropriate in this circumstance. I continued with my work, moving carefully and with deference to the fetus while contacting the spirit of the tumor. Extending the life force from my fingernails like tiny shovels instead of lasers, I effected the necessary micromanipulations that carefully gathered the tentacles of the tumor and coaxed it out of her body and into my hand, then on into the earth with a prayer for its transformation into its highest potential. I received reports throughout the rest of this pregnancy. After one week the grapefruit-sized tumor was reduced by half, and by the time she was ready to give birth it had disappeared completely. Rather than have the cesarean, she was able to deliver in a natural way at the hospital. Both mother and child were fine.

Over the years, I have done less and less actual psychic surgery in favor of more work with the totems, elements, and allies, or other Alchemical Healing methods. I find it more consistently effective to engage people in their own healing process rather than doing it for them. I have also learned that their imaginative visualizations and trance experiences are powerful opportunities for immediate changes to occur, and that healings that involve the patient in these ways have the advantage of being supported by continued work when I am no longer with them. (See Chapter 11, "Healing with Spirit Allies.")

THE SUCKING CURE

The very first shamanic healing that I witnessed was Rolling Thunder performing the sucking cure on Jerry Garcia, as related in Chapter 2. It was the event that inspired my interest in alternative healing, and throughout the years since, I have sought to understand what we experienced that day in 1969.

Subsequent research and travels have led me to realize that many indigenous shamanistic cultures have one or another version of the sucking cure. One of the shamans I work with in Peru uses a very direct form of this technique in his healing practice. He will often suck directly over the place where the symptom is located. He usually puts Auga de Florida or tobacco smoke in his mouth first for protection, and it is as though he is dancing with—as well as fighting with—the spirit. He then spits it out in a tissue or paper towel and continues doing so until the process is completed. Sometimes he vomits into a plastic bag, and, after the immediate part of the healing is complete, he will examine the contents of the bag to gain further information about the problem.

There was an incident that happened some years ago when I was working with him and tried to do a sucking cure his way. We were working with a woman who had a breast tumor. I neglected to use either tobacco or Florida Water when I attempted to suck out the spirit of the tumor directly, and I felt dangerously close to taking her problem into my own body. My shaman friend immediately sprayed me with the Florida Water, and my guide, Thoth, was somewhat severe in that moment when reminding me that this technique was not my way and that I should not be experimenting with it. I have necessarily become extremely cautious about working with any form of the sucking cure, and have determined that except for very rare and specific cases in which that seems the only appropriate alternative, I will not work with the direct sucking method at all.

The sucking cure that I will describe here is not a form that I recommend attempting unless you feel absolutely confident in your ability to keep yourself separate from that which you are removing.

And even then, be sure that your guidance is clear and that you trust where it is coming from. The sucking cure is one of the few arenas where there are strict rules that must be followed for your own safety. The first rule is: Don't swallow! That should be obvious, but I would not take it for granted in sharing this method.

My teacher for this healing technique is Sekhmet, the lioness-headed goddess of destruction and healing from Egypt. When I am preparing to work in this way, I invite her into my body, so as to access directly her ability to sniff out the original thought form at the source of the disease. She comes in as a lioness for this technique, and I can sometimes feel my nose wrinkle as she sniffs the person's head. This method of working with her also provides protection in what would otherwise place me in a situation where I would be more vulnerable than usual. It is as though she, Sekhmet, is using my body—my nose and my sense organs—in order to locate the problem. Then I begin to suck from the place where the pattern, the originating thought form of the disease or problem, is stored. I believe these patterns are held in the brain. I always approach through the crown chakra and leave it to Sekhmet to find the exact location from which to suck. When I am sucking, I am generally quite noisy, and I work with the sound and the breath in a variety of ways as I pull. Sometimes it's almost like kissing it out, very gentle and coaxing, and other times it requires all my strength.

It is important to maintain a conscious relationship with Sekhmet throughout the process, and I learn a great deal from her as she finds her way directly to the source of the problem. I can only do three or four passes, what I call the length of a full in breath; so each is carefully done and takes some time. Sometimes I hold the energy and take in more breath during a pass. I do not swallow, and at the apex of the breath I turn to spit, quite vociferously, into a bowl of water which has been placed to the side of where I am working. It is very important to get all remnants, physical and spiritual, out of your mouth each time, and into the water. Often I notice I am hissing or growling while these energies are being expelled.

In between each pass I check in with the person. Most everyone

I've worked with can distinguish whether and when things have loosened and are releasing when I am working with this method. Whether a very gentle drawing in is more effective, or a very strong one, I am coaxing the spirit of the problem all the while, until I know I have transferred everything into the water.

Because I will never suck more than four passes during any one healing, I must be careful with each time of sucking to get the most out of it, even allowing a breath or two while being extremely vigilant not to swallow or take anything into myself.

When the sucking has been completed, it is most important to refill lavishly. Sometimes I pour the element Water through the person, all the way through his body from the top of the head, to make sure all remnants that may have been shaken loose by this powerful technique are released from the body. You can have the person imagine he is sitting under a waterfall for a few moments to augment your use of Water.

When this form is used the crown chakra is opened during the process and must be gently closed at the conclusion of the work. This is accomplished with an upward motion of both hands, carefully bringing them almost together about eighteen inches to two feet above the head. This action helps to assure that the person is no longer vulnerable, as he might be if it were left open.

Any cleansing of this magnitude should be followed by a reminder to drink lots of water. If you can, give the person you are working on two glasses of water right away.

When the healing is complete, the bowl or jar of water that you used to receive the releases must be disposed of. It can be taken to a watercourse such as a river or stream that has outlet in the ocean or some other large body of water, or it can be offered to a tree, if permission is asked of the tree, or it can be buried in the earth. However you choose to dispose of it, you must do it with a prayer for its transformation into its highest potential. Your communication with the element or natural essence must be very clear, so that it will agree to hold the energies until they have transformed completely.

Once when I was working with a person who was experiencing

a psychotic break, we needed to leave the house we were in and move our work into another building. My attention was not on the water, and I left it in the first place where we started the healing. About half an hour later someone from the house came to get me to deal with the bowl of water I had left, because the family dog would not even enter the room where it stood.

CHOOSING YOUR METHODS

Recently, in Germany, I did separate private sessions on two people who suffer from migraines. On one person I did the sucking cure, and on the other I worked the Alchemical Healing formula with music. I chose my methods according to the needs of the moment, based on my sense of what each person was ready and willing to receive. Both healings were equally effective; however, to achieve that effectiveness, each needed to be done its own way.

There are many healing options, even in relation to the same symptoms. I choose one technique over another according to the guidance of the moment, my intuitive feeling about what is most appropriate, and my sense of what would be most powerfully received by the person requiring the healing.

Regardless of what form I use, communication enhances the experience. Many of my students who are clairvoyant or clairaudient can know for themselves what is going on and can tell when the healing is accomplished successfully. I can often feel it and have a knowing about the result. Sometimes it is not possible to communicate directly—when a person is in a coma, too young to speak, or perhaps speaks a different language. So it is best not to *need* to rely on communication, yet be able to avail yourself of the benefits when possible. So much of my healing work happens in the context of teaching and demonstrating that it is quite natural for me to work that way, and in so doing I have come to respect the advantages.

In your communications, ask the person what she is feeling. Tell her what you're feeling. Use your mind and trust your intuition. Go for what's practical and simple. Look for the path of least resistance.

Look within yourself to see who comes forward to help. Ask your client whom she sees. Share your feelings. Have fun. Trust your feelings. The energy itself has intelligence that you can rely upon as well. Pay attention.

Always remember, whichever method you employ in your healing work, you are conducting spirit, and you must do so with respect and without judgment. Nothing is intrinsically "bad," and all situations can be seen as opportunities for change. We can also honor our illness and injuries as our teachers. Regardless of how painful or inconvenient they are in our lives, they often force transformational changes that would otherwise not occur.

17
SOUND AND MUSIC

WHAT IS SOUND?

The subject of sound and music in healing is huge—actually a broad enough topic to fill its own book. In this chapter I offer an overview that contains some techniques, some principles, and, I hope, some revelations.

What is sound? Sound is the propagation of vibrational kinetic (movement) energy through some kind of matter, such as the atmosphere. The vibrations can vary through a wide range of frequencies (wave length). The lowest sound that we hear consists of a very slow frequency that can only be felt by our whole bodies, and the highest sound that we hear has a very fast frequency; beyond that high range are even faster, ultrasonic (beyond sound) frequencies our physical senses can't detect. We are aware of most of the frequencies between these two extremes through our hearing, but the effects of sound go well beyond what we can detect with our ears.

Everything in our physical reality is in a state of vibration. Vibration is movement between two poles, such as positive and negative, dense and rarified, being and nonbeing. A vibration occupies all states between these poles, except with sound there are actually no poles as stopping places, just phases of continuous movement. It is helpful to conceive of sound in these terms in order to explain how sound and music relate to healing. With sound there is a cyclical movement, a returning over and over again until the causal energy has become spent.

While in general terms, vibrations include all phenomena, sound itself is a specific range of frequencies that is attuned to the physical universe and the things in it. This does not mean that sound is purely physical, but rather, it is the most tangible way that all kinds of vibrational energies can interact and affect physical things. Everything in the universe is a vibration. It is more precise to say *a vibration* because it is necessary to honor the paradox that we cannot always say *what* is vibrating, or where the vibrations originate. It is the vibrations themselves, as energetic signatures, that we work with when using sound in Alchemical Healing. As sound makers, we have the ability to translate (or alchemize) a vast array of energies and intentions into sound and music by using our bodies, voices, and instruments to affect our surroundings.

Think of any thing, idea, or feeling, and imagine it as a vibration. It is important to realize that you are perceiving not just one frequency, like a dial tone, but that there are a plethora of vibrations that create that energetic signature. There is not just one frequency of love, for example, because love has many aspects. Love is a complex interrelationship of frequencies. This is one reason for the fact that what, why, who, or how the sound is made is of primary importance. Each way of making a sound creates a complex group of frequencies characteristic of the starting point of the sound. Some frequencies can be used for healing because they resemble and harmonize with the frequencies associated with the elements and energies used in Alchemical Healing.

Harmony and resonance are important principles in both music and healing. *Harmony* is the perception of a dynamic tension that is pleasant, when two or more frequencies blend together. These *consonances* (a fancy word for "pleasing sound") appear when the frequencies of the vibrations represent certain mathematical relationships. When we envision this as a form of sacred geometry, it illustrates the ways in which frequencies can work together creatively.

Resonance refers to what happens when a sound interacts with an object that tends to vibrate at a frequency that is in harmony with the sound. If you have a singing bowl, for instance, you can sing into it at the same pitch at which it rings, and it will begin to ring. Many instruments and objects will do this, which illustrates the point that sound can make an energetic connection between its source and an object. This principle is fundamental to how sound is used in healing, and with a little imagination you can see how this principle can be expanded to radically impact your healing work. When we listen to a song that opens the heart—we could even say that we have resonated with the song! This is an example of emotional resonance. The same emotional resonance can be duplicated through the healing energies we access in Alchemical Healing.

FINDING A SACRED INSTRUMENT

Finding a sacred instrument is like choosing a relationship. Forming a relationship with the instrument you choose, or the one that chooses you, is an important part of working with sound. It isn't really any different from forming a relationship with an animal totem, a plant spirit, or an element. If you already feel an affinity for one of the elementally associative instruments (described later), or if you have an intuition or impulse toward any particular instrument, then start your practice there. If not, but you feel drawn to the idea of exploring an instrument as a healing tool, you may wish to take a few moments to sit quietly and go inward to see which one to start with.

It is very conducive to healing to work with an instrument for which a specific purpose has been set through invocation and intention. The Stradivarius violins were crafted with the *conscious intention* of creating beautiful music. In many cultures drums are created with ceremony and intention, and are recognized to embody spirit. There is authenticity and power in what might appear to be a simple rattle, however the intention of its maker has a profound effect on the results of its use. I have seen stringed instruments, such as dulcimers and harps, that have been created with ritual and focused intention that set them apart as instruments of healing, beyond the beauty of the music they make.

Any instrument made *with the intention of healing* can be a powerful ally. For that reason, you may want to make your own instrument or to know something about the person who did make it.

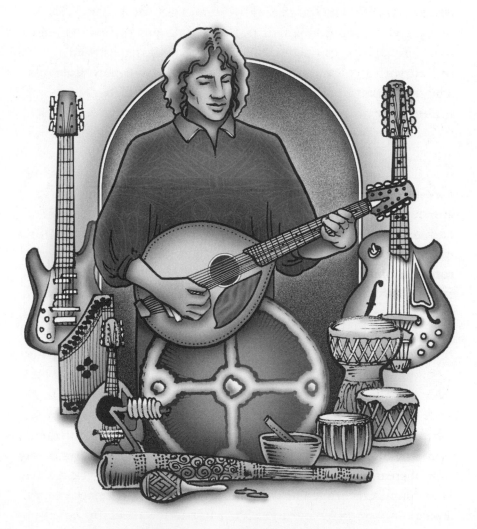

Figure 17.1. Sacred Instruments

When you are limited in what instruments are available at a given time, you may sensitively use whatever is at hand. For example, if you wish to heal with Water, you can ask a rattle (usually an Earth instrument) to hold the element of Water and to do a Water healing with you. It helps to have a well-developed relationship with that rattle and with the elements. You can always choose to *not* play an instrument, too, and can place it on your altar or in the room where you are doing the healing work and ask for its help. The rattle's presence would be a part of the healing process without actually being played, especially when you acknowledge its presence.

Totemic instruments are extremely precious and powerful blessings and should be honored as such. If an animal is dreamed or comes to you in a vision, and a related instrument comes in physical form, acknowledge that totem's energy. If the instrument is not already decorated, you can paint images or add physical decorations with intention that honor the totem in recognition of the gift. Follow your intuition; your gifts to your instrument and the decorations you put on it will help build your relationship with that instrument.

No matter how a sacred instrument comes into your possession, when there is resonance in your heart, it is wise to receive such a gift, unconditionally. Regardless of its humbleness, simplicity, or monetary value, it has called to you and the spirit of the instrument needs to be invoked and honored. There may be an unexpected gift, a request, or an instruction that will only come with your attention.

If you feel the impulse for your instrument to become a giveaway, pay attention and really check in about this. Sometimes this means your work is complete with this particular tool and it needs to be with someone else. Or perhaps you are being called to make space for a new instrument that is coming to you.

Know that you can also use whatever is available. Sometimes the right instrument is going to be a piece of wood, or a rock. I have made impromptu rattles by putting stones in empty water bottles. Sometimes you may be without your instrument, and it may call to you to be used in a particular healing. If this is so, use it! Imagine the instrument in your hand, honor its energetic presence, feel the energy signature that is that instrument's alone, and then go about the healing as though you actually have it in your possession.

When you know this, truly know this, you can go anywhere, anytime, be with or without your instruments, and still be effective with sound and vibrational healing. This is one of the ways that you can learn to honor your connection to the power and the energetic qualities of sound and vibrational healing.

SOUND PROTOCOL AND MANNERS

It is important to honor whatever specific instrument you are using, for when a musical instrument is created, the intention put into its creation enters into a life of its own, and a being results. Any serious musician knows this about her instruments, and it is equally important for you to understand that about any instrument you use for healing or ceremonial work. Invoke and honor the spirit of that instrument. Treat it as a ceremonial object. Also give it your intention and attention whenever you use it.

It is appropriate to say to your rattle, "I wish to access the healing wisdom of the stones for this healing." When you address the instrument as a conscious being, an ally, you greatly increase the effectiveness of its use as a healing tool. In some Native American traditions, the ceremonial instruments are smudged before they are used in a healing ceremony. Sometimes you will see the singer offer tobacco to the drum. When your work with your instrument is complete, remember to thank the instrument (along with any other help you have received, of course) for being your ally and for its help.

As with all sacred ritual objects, it is wise to ask if you may touch or play with someone else's healing instrument before picking it up. If that is not possible, ask with an open heart for permission from the instrument you wish to play. Even with your own instruments, it is good to be open-hearted enough to know when it is not appropriate to play, and when it is appropriate to allow or invite another to play your instrument.

Once you have consecrated an instrument for your use, be careful of how it is treated and into whose hands it falls. It is important to give it the same care you would a crystal that you have programmed, or a feather that you use in your healing work. And it is important to see that others do not mishandle it or treat it with disrespect.

PLAYING A SACRED INSTRUMENT

Relationships are developed through practice—in the case of instruments, through playing them. Start by making a practice of playing the instrument to yourself, and remaining absolutely present with the sound so that you get to know its various capabilities, learn the different kinds of sounds that it can make, and begin to gain an intuitive understanding of the instrument's energy signature. This will give you access into what those different sounds can accomplish or mean. As soon as you have achieved familiarity and an intuitive sense of your instrument, you must act on the intuitive insights to ground them and make them a part of your practice. For example, when I was in Peru, on the Amazon, I received a rattle that was decorated with carvings of the pink dolphins that dwell in the river there. When I journeyed using this rattle, it would change pitch for no apparent reason. Initially it was quite startling, but as I continued to pay close attention, I discovered a range of complexity that gradually became the language through which this rattle and I communicated. I could appreciate how those tonal changes were accenting moments of change in the journey, and I began to heed them for their insight.

Stay awake to the moment, and be responsible to what the moment is telling you. Pay attention to your body, and especially your heart, as you play the instrument. What is your posture? How do you feel? What gets tired? What gets energized? Are your eyes open or closed? When working with others it is important to keep your eyes open, so begin your practice with your eyes open at least half of the time. (Your eyes will become one of the ways that you can receive direct feedback on what you are doing, while you are doing it. Your sight will teach you how to read your clients' responses while they are having their experience.) Note any sensations or emotions that you feel in your body. This familiarity can guide you in a healing session, giving you a baseline bodily sense that allows you to notice when something is different, which could be valuable information. Use your instrument for that for which it is best suited as a tool, and remember that the intention is far more important than the execution. When it comes to playing, you must set aside any sense of good or bad, music played well or poorly, and really pay attention to what that instrument is asking you to play at that moment. The more you do it, the easier it will be, and in fact, the instrument will seem to play itself. That is the kind of relationship that you can develop with a healing instrument. If you are lucky enough to be able to train with or spend time with skilled sound healers, listen to their advice or teachings. But ultimately it is between you, spirit, and your clients. Once you know how to access this deeper level of vibrational healing, it no longer has to be your sacred rattle. It could be a cup with some rocks in it, or a jar with grains, beans, and rice. It can be someone else's instrument, or whatever happens to be at hand. The idea is to learn how to play in a way that accesses the healing nature of sound.

One of the hurdles that nearly everyone is going to have to face is what others think of their playing. Rationally, we know this is irrelevant—but that won't necessarily stop you from feeling self-conscious or self-critical. This again underscores the importance of playing the instrument for yourself, as a form of meditation during which you attune to the sound and how it feels in your body. The sound itself can be a profound teacher, for when you focus on the sound you are able to set aside your ego's perceptions and allow spirit to work through the body. Getting out of the way and developing your focus allows you to be more present and spontaneous with your playing. A happy consequence of this practice is that your awareness will begin to expand. You will naturally become more aware of the sonic needs of the people you are working with. By allowing this awareness to develop, over time, you will become more grounded and effective in your work.

You can also begin to experiment with the different types of sounds you can make, how those different types of sounds that the instrument makes might affect you, which organs they can affect, and what kind of emotional imprints might be present. Notice which sounds make it easier or more difficult to remain focused. This last one is significant for any journey work that you wish to do with your instrument. Journey work requires that the music or sound hold the focus without being a distraction and without allowing distraction. All instruments can do this. Our definition of *instrument* is anything that produces sound. It is meaningful when considering all the sources of sound that are available to you, to consider the range of sounds and the ability and responsiveness of the instrument. The sound that is generated when I tap on this keyboard would have limited applications compared with a rattle or drum. To catalyze meditative journey work, one must be skilled and attuned to the spirit of vibrational healing, the elements, one's higher self, and the instrument. And to achieve this state of attunement, one must remember that spirit is conducting the dance between musician and the meditation.

INSTRUMENTS AND THE ELEMENTS

For most of us, musical instruments are imbued with an energetic presence—especially those that are or have been used ceremonially. If you choose to use such instruments and you take the time to get to know their energetic presence, that knowledge will be helpful in determining what instrument to use at any given time. Some have a native element, one with which they have special affinity. Often this is due to the way the sound is created within the instrument, who made the instrument, or how it was made. All the elements have a characteristic vibratory quality, so even though Water is most visibly wavelike, this wavelike quality is present in all elements, although in the case of Akasha it is mysterious, beyond descriptions or words.

Instruments are said to have an affinity for a particular element, but none is a "pure" embodiment of that element. Each instrument also has aspects that do not relate to its primary element.

- The rattle is a sound of the Earth element. The rattle is associated with Earth for the simple reason that it is the stones in the rattle that speak. Rattles are not always filled with stones, of course, but generally the Earth element is connected to the lowest frequencies—fundamental tones—and rhythms. It is about how we walk on the earth and what is experientially tangible and real.

- The sound of the drum radiates out in waves and is associated with the element Water. The drum's mode of vibration is associated with Water because it is a vibrating surface—an edge or interface between things. It is associated with the loving heart because it symbolizes the interface between spirit and matter. It is the realm of pure (and purifying) frequencies of the middle range of human hearing.

- The flute and the human voice conjure Air. Air, because if its elasticity and freedom of movement, is about pure harmonies and harmonics and occupies the highest frequency range. Its aspects are clarity and understanding. Instruments that employ a mechanism of exciting air to the point of vibration are affiliated with this element—flutes, whistles, the voice.

- The sistrum, cymbals, and gongs convey the sound of Fire. The Fire element is associated with chaos—the breakdown of order and structure—and with the transformative process. Fire sounds occupy the entire sound frequency range because they include all the unpitched and extremely complex sounds—cymbals, gongs, breaking glass, firecrackers, and so forth.

To remember the primary elemental associations, imagine the stones or pebbles speaking in the rattle; the surface of a drum like the rippling surface of water; air moving through the flute; the chaos of the cymbals and the fire that forged them.

Most instruments blend the elements. The drum, for example, speaks in all the elements—Fire because impact transforms the quiescent drum into a vibrating instrument, Water because the drum's membrane vibrates in waves, Air because the membrane excites the air next to it to vibration, and Earth because just one hit makes a fundamental tone, and because the drum's rhythmic beat reflects the heartbeat of the earth. But it is the vibrating membrane that defines it as a drum, as opposed to some other instrument, so that definitive characteristic establishes the drum's primary relationship with Water.

These affinities are not so much about a relationship between an element and an instrument, as they are about a relationship between an element and a way of making sound. Instruments employ certain ways of making sound, which establish the affinities. Understanding these "ways of making sound" contributes to an ability to use the elements with sound.

If you wanted to work with Water and Air, you could use a guitar or another stringed instrument, because strings combine those elements. Bass guitars strike the lowest frequencies of Water, which are associated with the libido, creation, and sex. These low frequencies reach to our deepest longings as animals, and sexual drive is very much a part of those longings.

These are merely a few general examples. As you make your relationship with your instrument, you can work with it to find its many elemental voices.

The fifth element, Akasha, is associated with and represented by the spaces between, and the interims of, sound—the sound of silence, ambience, and reverberation. It is a difficult and advanced technique to access the Akasha of sound, yet it is available for one who is aware of the subtle qualities of ambient sound. In a church, if you make a loud sound, there is a great deal of ambience, or reverberation, yet this ambience exists no matter where you are. You will find it in a forest, in a room, on a lake, and so on. Each environment will present reflective surfaces (or not) that affect the sound environment of that space, as well as having ambient or incidental sounds that exist in that space. Akasha is the void from which form emerges, and is also a storehouse of all the information in the universe. Because of this, incidental or random sounds can be interpreted as feedback or hints from the universal mind. This urges us to expand our awareness to be more inclusive, and to be mindful in our healing practice.

When you are working with Akasha, it is important to consider the room from an acoustic standpoint, in other words, how sounds *sound* in the room. Generally, uneven surfaces and a mix of hard and soft surfaces will yield the most flexible sound environments—sounds made in such environments may be reverberated, but not significantly altered. In many of the ancient traditions around temples and cathedrals, it is said that one can hear the words of the gods in the sounds between the sounds. If you look at the interior of such places, you will see complex surfaces (no flat walls) and a mixture of soft and hard surfaces. Such spaces are suitable for all kinds of sound work. There are also acoustic spaces that resonate in specific ways. They are usually characterized by being resonant in certain frequencies (and not in others) or will have "focal points" where sound is concentrated. There are numerous ancient sites designed to this purpose, as well. The choice to use this kind of acoustic space in your own work should be made with sensitivity and experience as the effect they have on sound work can be very powerful.

THE HUMAN VOICE

The human voice is perhaps the most versatile musical instrument. Ironically, it is both the most difficult and the easiest to use. Words and language are things that other instruments cannot contain. If you intend to use your voice in the capacity of healing, meditation, or journey, you must be aware of the effect of words, as well as how you speak or sing the words. If voice is to be your instrument, you must understand how prayer, chants, poetry, mantras, and invocations affect the relaxed psyche of the meditative journeyer, for these are designed to go beyond mere communication, and this aspect of spoken language is beyond the scope of this chapter.

What is within the scope of this chapter is using the voice as a toning tool. The voice can be used for journey and trance work, as other instruments can. The human voice is unique when toning in that it does not embody any of the elements, and embodies all of them. First and foremost, it embodies us as spirit-infused animals. It is the Air of spirit that allows the human voice to sound; yet all of the elements are involved. If you wish to work with your voice in this way, you must practice on yourself. Although it is difficult to listen to your own singing or vocalizations, you can do it. As with any instrument, allow your attention to focus in your body and pay attention to what changes happen in your body when you are making the sounds. If the sound grows louder in volume, there should be a corresponding sensation in some part of your body.

To use the voice as a healing instrument is an advanced practice. Yet it can be cultivated with respect for the great power that is brought into play. I was taught to simply open and receive the appropriate tone for the moment, and to then release it from a place deep inside of me. The results were often measurable, as in the following experience, which happened when I first learned of the concept. Subsequent experiments indicated that the vibratory frequencies emitted through toning could change the fabric of reality. Thus, they should be used in a mindful way and with caution.

GRANDPA ROBERTS

Shortly after I was introduced to the concept of healing with sound, I was visiting the herb school on my land in California. Grandpa Roberts, an elder who was living in a pod in the hills there, was a healer and medicine person, and he expressed interest in what I was learning about sound. He asked me to work on an arrhythmia problem he was having with his heart. Forty-nine years earlier he had been bitten by a black widow spider. He went into a coma and was momentarily mistaken for dead, but at the hospital, he suddenly sat up and looked around. Ever since then he had suffered from a stuck heart valve that caused heart palpitations in an ongoing cycle: after a certain pattern of beats, the pressure would build and create pain as the cycle completed, and the scenario would begin again. I was a little taken aback when he suggested I work on this longstanding chronic problem, but I took it on as an interesting challenge.

I started with basic alchemical energy work and made a strong connection. When I intuited that a sound wanted to come through, I became very clear and focused, took a deep breath while asking inwardly for just the right tone to come through, and released a sound—a tone that seemed to pierce the veil between spirit and matter. It wasn't that it was particularly loud, but it was certainly penetrating. The tone was still emanating when Grandpa Roberts became extremely excited. He started speaking so fast I could not understand what he was saying. I finally realized that he was describing a journey he was spontaneously taking through his blood stream.

When he was done he gave me a great hug and exclaimed that he was cured: from the moment the tone had started, the valve that had been caught slipped into place, relieving all symptoms instantly. Then, to his additional amazement, he was treated to a tour of his circulatory system and his heart.

SILENT SOUND

There are times when, though the use of sound in a healing is called for, it is inappropriate for you as healer to call attention to what you are doing. Please understand that whatever frequencies you can send out in an auditory manner can also be sent out silently. When I was first introduced to this concept, the skeptic within me jumped up and made lots of noise. Naturally, I had to try it. My first experience doing a healing using silent sound was also done by telephone, with a friend who was suffering from a debilitating migraine headache. This was a chronic problem for her, and nothing she had discovered had yet given her anything but minimal and temporary relief.

After discussing the details of her plight, I suggested that she pay close attention while I aimed a silent tone directly (through the phone lines) to the point in her head where the pain was greatest.

As I inhaled, I asked for the perfect tone to be brought into being, and my intention was extremely focused as I conveyed the tone that came up, silently, into the phone. Immediately a large black spider came into Christine's inner vision, right at the base of her head where the point of pain was greatest. The spider had a grip on her head, and the tone was shaking it, as if to dislodge the spider from its tight hold. Every time I would create the tone, the spider would begin to discorporate, and the pain would diminish. When I stopped, it became solid again, but to a lesser degree each time, until the pain was relieved and the spider finally disappeared. Meanwhile, Christine was receiving an understanding of her personal process. Her chronic migraines, according to this experience, were the result of continually stuffing truth to avoid conflict. In so doing, she was feeding the symbolic spider, and when it grew large enough its presence would ignite the migraine.

Healings of this nature, where a person is given a clear indication regarding cause and effect, are sustained according to the person's willingness to change the offending pattern of behavior.

SACRED SONGS AND CHANTS

It is advantageous to recognize the power of sacred sound and especially rhythm, for it is the preferred conveyance of shamans throughout time, regardless of whether they use sacred plant medicines or not. For those who use sacraments, sound is a vital component and functions as a vehicle to achieve the intention of the shamans and the attention of their allies. Certain rhythms have certain effects on the body and psyche, and any study of shamanism throughout the world will reveal that these rhythms are incorporated in their songs, chants, and ceremonies, and especially their healing work.

The voice can be used, with the appropriate intention, with a chant that has been carefully learned and practiced. These chants or songs have a life of their own, a special relationship in consciousness. When you sing a specific chant or song, you are asking for the help of the energy and spirit of the song. And so it is very important that you know what the energy is. Alternatively, if a song, chant, or melody comes to you, especially in healing work or in ceremony, you can safely accept the gift. Realize that it is up to you to understand what that gift can be used for. Usually you will know at the time you receive it.

Songs are like instruments in that they have consciousness. As conscious beings, they should be treated with respect, and there are some songs that you must receive specific permission to use. If you receive a song that you know is a sacred or healing song, in some way other than from a teacher who is authorized to give you that song, it is important to be very careful in using it. With an open heart, ask for its permission. And be quite prepared to hear a "No." Some songs are powerful allies that have been held sacred for many, many generations. The traditions of these songs must be honored and respected; if not, the songs get changed, and the sacred power within the songs, in turn, changes. It is possible that you could be gifted with a song, especially if you intuit that a song is needed and you request one.

HEALING WITH SOUND AND MUSIC

Those who find it difficult to heal with the hands may have a better experience with healing through sound and music, and of course these methods can be used together. You will know if sound is to be one of your tools. Yet even if it is not, you must cultivate an awareness of sound and how it affects the healing process. The sounds that surround us on a daily basis can have a profound effect on people. Sometimes it is necessary to ask someone to remove himself from a certain sound environment or put himself into a certain sound environment in order for healing to take place. You may wish to investigate the possibility of staging your healings at a specific place, like at the beach, along a stream, at certain concerts, or even during a thunderstorm. The key, as always, is to be openhearted as to whether it is the right thing—and completely unattached to the answer. This discernment is a skill that often requires development.

For healing purposes we draw a distinction between sound and music that looks like this: music is something that was composed or recorded prior to its use, while what we are calling sound is something created spontaneously, on the spot. It may be that this sound is rhythmic or melodic, yet we call it sound because, in the moment of its creation, all its attributes are alive to everything that's happening at that moment. Some forms of music, such as chants and healing songs, can behave in this way too, and so are a bit of both— sound and music—because they were composed before the fact.

CHOOSING MUSIC

Music, along with visual arts and other art forms, provides us with a vital opportunity to combine basic alchemical physics with the cultural aspect of being human. A healer will develop sensitivity to the cultural meaning for music in general, and also for a particular piece of music. By *cultural*, I mean all of our ways that we received from our parents and the human world around us; this includes concerns about our personal identity, most of our emotions, and certainly many of our fears.

Using music, such as a recorded CD, for healing is a very different discipline than working with pure sound. It requires you to look more deeply at the meaning and intention of any piece of music you choose to work with. Your understanding can be arrived at both logically and intuitively. The point is that music brings with it a layer of intention, tradition, and meaning that come from outside the room, and thus it requires that you understand just what you are bringing in. Sound, for the most part, lacks this extra layer of complexity.

That said, I have noticed that whatever piece of music I choose seems to work with me, and often I don't know what I'm dealing with until I get into the healing work. I have worked with trance/dance, rock and roll, Gregorian and other sacred chants, classical music, world fusion, and drums. There are times when I have to work with whatever I am given, if, for example, I find myself doing healing work at a concert or a restaurant. One of the mysteries I've encountered is that the music will resonate with whatever I'm doing. As if by magic, the flute starts as I call on Air or the drummer hits the cymbal when I invoke Fire. When I am familiar with a particular CD I can work with the elemental energies that I know are there. I suppose there could be situations where that would not be the case; however, in my personal experience I have always been able to work with and find power to assist me in the music.

EMOTIONAL HEALING AND MUSIC

Music, because of its relationship to emotions, can be a very effective tool if you understand what it is that you are trying to do. For instance, if you are doing healing work with someone and realize that anger is causing disease, you may find it effective to use angry music to allow that person to see and know her own anger and perhaps even help her to express it. This is to be distinguished from indulging in anger. You will know the difference by the catharsis process—the transformation of the emotion is very clear when it is cathartic in nature, although in Alchemical Healing catharsis is rarely necessary.

All emotions are actually love in different forms, so when emotions transform, they are moving toward love, toward becoming an emotion of love. The emphasis is on the words *toward* and *transformation*. Transformation cannot occur in the presence of indulgence. It cannot occur in people who have created a feedback loop with their emotions, because when you cling to emotions, they will not transform. They may subside; but subsiding is different from transforming. For an emotion to merely stop being an issue for the moment is not necessarily a healing process. The distinction is significant because the transforming of emotion is fundamental to the healing process. When an emotion goes through a transformation, healing occurs.

In fact, the transformation of an emotion is a hallmark of healing. For example, fear may turn to anger because fear is at the opposite pole of love, and anger is a step closer to love. When fear turns to anger, it is a movement toward love and an opportunity to honor yourself with love. You may attempt to go directly from fear to love. Or anger might transform into grief, bringing things a little closer to love, and closer to an opening of the heart.

Although anger might transform to sorrow, grief, or directly into love, the important thing is to know the difference between an emotion transforming, and an emotion simply stopping. The ways that emotions are stopped are that they are buried, or that they run out of energy to be expressed. Under either of these circumstances, the emotion of anger will continue to be present and continue to do whatever it does. Halting the grieving process may result in depression, while allowing it to proceed and transform naturally into joy permits healing to occur around the loss.

Remember to resist the temptation to counteract an emotion with its opposite. For example, attempting to use a joyful piece of music when you are working with grief might not be as effective as finding music that supports the grief. Look for music that can be a supportive container, and use that music to create a space where the emotion is empowered to transform.

Music is a powerful way to catalyze feelings. It can create a space for emotions to transform by being a container where permission is given to feel the emotion. Skilled composers can consciously stimulate emotions when they create music. Often they are expressing what they are feeling, and the music embodies that. They have placed their intention, perhaps for their own healing or emotional expression, into a piece of music, and when you then use that music for healing, this intention is available to the healing process.

The first step to healing an emotion is often to create a space for it to be okay to feel that emotion, especially regarding feelings and emotions that are frowned upon in a cultural context. People need to know that they are not their emotions, that emotion is an energy—one of the many energies that reside within them—and that energy can be allowed to flow without consuming the whole being. Because emotions ebb and flow, when they are allowed to flow they will ebb soon after. Music is an extremely potent tool for creating a space of acceptance for this flow.

It is important to know your tools: to know what they are capable of, to really know what the intention is that went into them. You can know that intuitively. If the intention is to make money, you will know it. A song written with that sole intention will not be of much use. That is not to say that a songwriter that needs to make money cannot write a good healing song. As always, the intention is more important than just about anything. When you use music for healing you must know or trust the intention that went into that music.

EXERCISES FOR DEVELOPING SOUND HEALING TOOLS AND TECHNIQUES

Here are some exercises to help develop your sound healing tools. The first is the basic practice for using an instrument intentionally.

EXERCISE
Intentional Sound

Find a comfortable, quiet spot to play your instrument. Pick an intention to invoke, such as calming, relaxation, Water movement, or Fire burning.

Focus your attention on your breath.

Hold your intention in your mind—visualize it, internally chant it, or just state the intention, speaking it out loud or internally. Keep holding your focus on your breath as you do this.

Now release the invocation and allow your instrument to speak into this space, just letting the sound express itself as it wants to. Don't think about what it should sound like; don't try to be descriptive with the sound; just let it intuitively happen.

Listen while you play—focus your attention on the *sound,* not on your playing. This will take a little practice, but it is the key to building an intuitive relationship with the instrument. Let your body do the playing without the mind directing it, occupying the mind with the listening.

As you practice this, look for sounds that help hold the focus of the intention. If you find yourself distracted, return your attention to the sound of the instrument, hearing every detail, following the sound like the words of a story. You may develop sounds that go with a specific intention that you will use every time you wish to invoke that intention—or maybe it will be different each time. The point of the exercise is to put your conscious control of the instrument aside and let your body, and the intention, play the instrument.

All instruments are capable of focusing sound to a specific part of the body or energetic field. This can be done with the intention in a way similar to the above exercise, by sending the instrument's energy to a specific spot without actually moving the instrument to that spot. Some instruments lend themselves to being positioned or directed. Rattles and sistrums can direct energy in this way easily. Singing bowls can be placed on the body and played. Wind instruments can direct a powerful stream of energy and should be used with some caution, especially the didgeridoo. Seek instruction before using a "didge" directly on someone's body. It is much safer to point it *around* the body, where it can still move an amazing amount of energy.

Focusing Sound

This exercise is simple to experiment with and requires a partner. Ask your partner to give you feedback of any feelings or sensations he might have as you direct different sounds to different parts of the body and also around the body. Don't be discouraged if the effects are subtle or unnoticeable; you will be developing a familiarity by using your instrument in this way. Bring your observations from your individual practice to these experiments, as you may have noticed certain frequencies or sounds affecting certain parts of your body as you play.

Know that these directed sounds do not only affect the physical body, but they also affect all the body's energetic fields. For safety as well as for the most profound effect, you must have your intention, your attention, and your relationship with the instrument developed especially in order to maintain the subtlety required to do healings on higher energetic levels. The physical level is a lot more accessible.

Elemental Invocation

This powerful practice is best done with four people and four instruments. It can be done alone, with one instrument connecting to each of the four elements.

Bring in each element one by one, then bring in Akasha with your attention: this means you must listen to what the room, or trees, or mountain is throwing back at you, listening to the space. The invocation allows for each person with an instrument to invoke the element, that element's qualities, and to play the instrument . . . then stop. It is essential to hold a moment of silence at each stop: that silence is what contains the gift. It may not be something you recognize consciously. Nevertheless, hold your mind silent at that moment. The sound of the instrument will help you focus on the sound that spirit, or the space, will send back to you when the instrument has stopped. This is one way to invoke Akasha.

Now add a powerful final invocation of Akasha by playing all four instruments at the same time, then stopping all at once, letting the reverberation be the voice of Akasha. There is power in the resulting cacophony, so go for it! And then let the silence speak. . . .

Silence is what defines the sound and the rhythm. It is what contains the healing opportunities and the realization of unmanifest dreams. Learning to dance between the notes and the silence is the true training ground of the soul's ability to embody sound as a healing modality.

18
SELF-HEALING

HEALING THE HEALER

My life changed dramatically when I started practicing healing. It was in retrospect that I discovered the source of the improvement in the quality of my life. Not only did I have more energy as a result of generating energy in this way, there were some unexpected side benefits: I naturally abandoned certain unhealthy aspects of my lifestyle because of the influence they would have on the recipients of the healing energies. Although the changes were gradual, it has become a matter of self-respect that I strive to maintain a strong, healthy body and emotional equanimity.

It has been my observation that many gifted healers withhold their newly learned skills due to timidity or lack of confidence. It has also been my observation that whenever they overcome their self-imposed barriers these tentative healers are rewarded with the little successes that encourage them to expand their practices. This world is in such need that I would advise you to put aside your reservations. Whether or not you have already realized it, you are capable at this moment.

In a sense, every time we attempt to heal another, we are also healing ourselves. Although you generally receive energy as a result of giving it, there are times when you need to maintain boundaries in order to assure your own health. When you are recovering from illness or injury yourself, you have to make that determination with care, according to an honest self-assessment and perhaps a check-in with your spirit guides.

Any and all of the techniques and practices that you can perform on another person, you can do for yourself too (except, of course, the obvious, such as the sucking cure). The easiest and most commonly used self-healing tool is a simple laying on of hands, which can be done at any time, though an especially good time to do it is when you are just about to go to sleep. Try placing your hands on or directing them to the place of need; turn the energy on; and then, when you have a good flow going, allow yourself to fall asleep. The energy will keep running until the place of need is filled.

That being said, I prefer other healers working on me whenever possible. It took an interesting situation, however, to realize how much power we have over our own healing process when we apply the more sophisticated tools of Alchemical Healing to our own needs.

HEALING A COLD SORE

I was about to be interviewed on the radio in San Francisco, my first interview ever, live. Quite nervous and stressed, I had just driven down from Oregon with little time to spare. It was less than an hour before I was due at the radio station, and while I was getting dressed at a friend's home, I felt the familiar sensation of a herpes blister about to break out on my upper lip. I knew that once it broke the skin it would hurt like crazy, I would not be able to smile, and it would affect my speaking.

I stopped what I was doing to give full attention to the rapidly developing situation, and was able to connect easily, feeling the energy quite clearly. I used my right fingers to make a laser incision right over (about two inches above) the burgeoning blister, opened it up to gain access, then poured gentle energy into the area. I then called on the plant cayenne, the plant I know to be most effective for the relief of herpes. I offered a blast of energy to its family, then waited to feel the etheric substance of the cayenne coalesce in my hand. As I directed the cayenne into the blistered area, I was surprised that it felt cool rather than warm. After a short wait, I began to pull at the blister as though my hand were a magnet, offering the aka that I gathered to the earth, then repeating the process several times. I refilled the space with liberal amounts of energy, with additional cayenne included.

The entire process took less than twenty minutes, and the relief was immediate. By the time I left for the radio station there was no sign of the attack, and it did not return.

THE HEART BREATH

There are certain Alchemical Healing techniques that you can do for yourself that you cannot do for anyone else. Breathing exercises are among the techniques that are extremely potent for self-healing. Eastern yoga techniques rely on the harmonization of the breath with the physical postures, to aid in the body's nourishment and flexibility. As is true for any meditative discipline, Alchemical Healing is enhanced by disciplined breath control. Control of the breath leads to mastery; directing the breath consciously helps to fine-tune subtle energies, as we have seen in the Caduceus Empowerment.

We influence the world around us simply by breathing. And we can learn a lot about ourselves and others by paying attention to the breath. I recommend incorporating breath practices from other systems into your practice of Alchemical Healing whenever possible. The Heart Breath practice that follows can be incorporated into your healing practice, and your daily life, with great benefit. During the first year of my studies with Nadia, she taught us how to journey into the elemental kingdoms to learn directly from the elements themselves. Nadia tended to be somewhat secretive with the teachings; however, during a particular exercise, we were told that whatever we were given we would be free to incorporate into our practices and to share with others. It was during an Akashic adventure that I was first shown the possibility that we are transformers, in a literal way. We have the capacity to take toxins, pollution, and angst into our bodies and transform them into love, a form of nourishment that we can then express back out into the world. When I returned from my journey, Nadia responded to my sharing with some surprise. "Yes," she said. "This is most certainly possible. However, it is an advanced technique and I strongly suggest that you wait for some time before you begin that practice."

Many years later, some others and I were working with Peruvian shamans who taught us about the concept of *ayne,* the principle of reciprocation inherent to the Incan and Quechuan, or pre-Incan, ways of life. Along the banks of the river that flows through Aguas Caliente and along the base of Machu Picchu there are many boulders, worn round by the turbulence of the rushing waters. We took some time to climb along the river, making a ceremony of gratitude and practicing new healing techniques we were being shown by our shaman guides. In that place we were taught a breath that is intended to be used consciously to give back to Pachamama, our Mother Earth. I was reminded then of my initial journey to Akasha and was prompted to adapt what the Peruvians showed me into what I now call the Heart Breath.

The Heart Breath is a powerful step in developing ourselves as transformers. It is the nature of breath to carry whatever intention is expressed in the moment, in a way similar to the way it carries the scent of the one that is breathing. When you practice the Heart Breath, the intention is most potently developed during the inbreath, the inspiration. The power gathers at the apex of the breath, that moment when the breath has been inhaled and before it is released intentionally during the exhale. Once the energies of above and below converge and mingle with the fire in your heart, the exhale will carry your intention with the love energy from the heart out into the world.

Practicing the Heart Breath cultivates the felt experience of sustaining a presence in the heart center. This breath can be used to rekindle your own heart flame as well as to transform your current emotions, feelings, and ambient surroundings into the energies of love and compassion. For our purposes in learning the following exercise, simply focus on your breath, allowing yourself to experience the movement of the breath into and out of your body as described. We will incorporate this into other practices as we delve more deeply into self-healing through Alchemical Healing.

EXERCISE
Heart Breath

Be sure to ground and center yourself before beginning to practice the Heart Breath. . . .

Once you feel grounded and centered, begin by drawing your breath as though you were pulling it up from deep within the earth. While you intend the movement of your breath, focus on it and feel as the breath moves up through your body to the level of your heart center. . . .

Let the breath mingle for a moment with your inner heart flame . . . then exhale with the intention of sending your breath out through your heart center and into the world.

Breathe in that way for a few breaths. . . .

Now bring your attention to the sky above you, and intend to draw your breath from above, as though you were pulling it down from the sky. Feel it flow into your body through your crown as you draw it down to the level of your heart, again allowing it to mingle for a moment with the flame in your heart center. . . . Now exhale with the intention of sending your breath out through your heart center and into the world.

Do this breath several times. . . .

Now draw the breath from the earth and sky simultaneously,

and experience the two breaths coalesce at your heart flame for a moment before you send it out into the world. . . .

Continue to breathe in this manner—in from above and below at the same time, gathering in your heart, and expressing out into the world as love.

The Heart Breath can be incorporated into your daily activities as well as your spiritual practices. You will know that you are in alignment with your heart center when you are aware of the fullness of being, the hugeness of the creation and your integral place in it, and the deep compassion and love you feel for all life—and particularly for those around you. Self-absorption simply vanishes in the light of the perfection of the moment, and you become receptive to inspiration beyond your personal imaginings.

BREATHING THE ELEMENTS

Breathing the elements consciously—one of the most powerful self-healing techniques—requires more care than working the elements with your hands. Drawing the symbol in the air and running the energy through your hands utilizes a more subtle level of the elements than breathing them into yourself. Breathing the elements is stronger because on your breath the elements are closer to the form in which they manifest in matter. Akasha is not used in these exercises, because of its volatile nature.

There are two ways of breathing with the elements. The first, Pulse Breathing, involves breathing directly to specific organs or parts of your body that require special attention, such as injured, diseased, or stressed areas. The second allows you to breathe elements directly into your body through your pores. It must be noted that because of the strength of the elements when breathed, at no time should you direct elements to the heart or the brain.

PULSE BREATHING

Every part of the body functions in rhythm. Life is constantly pulsing in and out of existence at various rates. From the largest organs to the smallest cells and molecules, the frequency with which each particle comes in and out of form creates a tone, a vibration. When everything resonates in harmony, there is health, and when a person or part of a person is out of tune, when there is dissonance in the body, illness occurs.

You have the capacity to focus upon and perceive the rhythm of any part of your body. The heartbeat provides the most obvious example, because we all can feel it. The pulses that you take at your wrist provide a subtler example. Most of us can feel the main pulse of the blood moving through our veins; however, it requires even deeper attention and training to distinguish the more subtle pulses that provide diagnostic information for Chinese acupuncture practitioners. These pulses relate to the energy currents associated with the organs, which are also found at the wrists. Focused attention upon any part of your body will yield its pulse, the rhythm created by the congregation of energy in motion. Directing elements through breathing is done by synchronizing your breath to the rhythms of your body.

For example, let's say your kidneys show symptoms of stress. You can place your hands on your back or aim them to direct energy. You can make the Water symbol and connect with Water to flush your kidneys. These same healing energies are certainly what you might choose to do for others with similar complaints.

For yourself, however, it is stronger to breathe the element of choice directly to the organ. To do this, you focus on your kidney until you find its pulse. Then you synchronize your breathing until you feel yourself in resonance with the pulse of your kidney. As you slow your breathing you will feel the pulse of your kidney slow as well. Now you can release the element directly into the kidney through the resonance you have created with its pulse. As mentioned above, in this case, you would choose Water to flush your kidneys.

Again, do not send these energies directly to the heart or brain.

PORE BREATHING

The second form of self-healing with the elements is accomplished through pore breathing. The largest organ of the human body is the skin, which is an eliminatory system that functions to release toxins from the body. When you learn to utilize the pores as a two-way access, you can very quickly achieve effects that might take considerably longer by other methods. You accomplish this access by synchronizing your breath with the pulse of your pores. Because the rhythm of the pores is so quick, you must syncopate the rhythms by pacing your breathing: speed it up for a moment to connect with the rhythms of your pores; then slow down your breath, and the rhythms of your pores will slow down so that you can breathe the element directly into your body through your pores. You can call certain powers or aspects of the element in with your breath, and you can remove those aspects of the element that don't serve your purpose at the final part of the exercise.

As with all the other organs and parts of our bodies, our pores have rhythms that we can connect to and resonate with. Once you learn to find and establish resonance with that rhythm, you can begin to draw elements into your body, filling it quite rapidly with the element of choice. It is necessary, while inhaling the element, to focus your attention on the aspect or quality of the element that you want to utilize. For example, if you are feeling fear and need courage for whatever reason, you might choose an infusion of Fire, because courage is an aspect of Fire. There are many aspects of Fire, and it is possible to want to draw in some aspects while at the same time avoiding others.

Pore breathing requires you to distinguish between the *power* of the element and the element itself. The power to affect transformation comes from the essence of the elements, and you must always release the actual element from wherever you've directed it as soon as it has been held long enough to impart its essence. The power remains in the essence that has been left behind, in direct relationship with your intention. Because of the strength, when you breathe in the elements through your pores you must take care not to accumulate them any longer than necessary for the transfer. Remember, although you are drawing these energies into your entire body, do not accumulate them in your heart or brain.

It's helpful to have a good working knowledge of the elements and the various aspects of each before practicing this breath work. Following is an exercise that will help you to comprehend the power of pore breathing.

EXERCISE
Balancing the Elements in Your Body

This exercise in pore breathing is used to harmonize the elements in your body. It is effective when you are about to face difficult situations such as the sweat lodge, extreme weather, physical trial, or any condition where you need extra balance. You can use it to restore the balance of the elements when you feel off center or elementally out of kilter.

Relax, ground, and center. . . . Concentrate on seeing yourself as an empty vessel, the receptacle that you are. The outer edges of your vessel are shimmering. As you continue to concentrate, the shimmering takes on a rhythm as you connect to the pulse of your pores. Focus on the pulse of your pores, and synchronize your breath with that pulse. You cannot breathe that fast, but you can find the resonance where the two rhythms fit together, like a high drum and a low drum playing fast and slow rhythms that fit together into a synchronized whole. . . . When you now slow down your breathing, the pulse of your pores will slow down also. . . .

Now begin to breathe Earth into your body, from your feet to the base of your spine, filling that part of your body with the element Earth. . . .

When the lower part of your body is filled with Earth, begin to fill the middle part, from the base of your spine to your ribcage, including your entire abdominal region, with the element Water. Because you are pulling the element in through your pores, it will fill rapidly and you will be able to notice the difference between how those two parts of your body feel. . . .

Next breathe Air into your chest and arms, including your throat. Fill the upper part of your body with Air and feel the quality of that element in your body. . . .

When you have taken in all the Air that part of your body can hold, concentrate on breathing in Fire to your head. It will quickly fill. Then breathe slowly for a moment, holding all four elements in your body, and knowing that these elements are working to balance your body elementally. . . .

After a short time, a minute or two at most—you will have an instinctive knowledge of when it is complete—begin to release, first the Fire from your head with each outbreath. When that is totally released, breathe out the Air from your upper torso and arms. Then exhale the Water from your abdominal region and finally the Earth from your lower body.

It is imperative to release fully each element, because it is not safe to hold the gross elements in your body. Their power remains after the interaction of the elements with your physical body and with your intention is complete.

Disconnect your attention from the elements and breathe normally. Notice how it feels to be balanced in this way.

CHANGING YOUR CHARACTER

Pore breathing the elements can dramatically change one's personality when done with appropriate intention. The following technique is an excellent way to begin to understand the elements, while doing some powerful work on yourself. If you are vigilant in your practice, you should see impressive results within three months. The object of this work is to begin to view yourself elementally and to restructure your character by changing the balance of the elements within yourself.

On a piece of paper, make two lists in two columns. On the left, list all the things that you like about yourself. Look at each of the qualities that you have listed, and determine which element relates strongly to that attribute. Draw the symbol of the element next to the quality. Some characteristics may relate to more than one element.

In the right-hand column, make a list of all the things that you *don't* like about yourself, and look at those characteristics elementally, drawing the appropriate symbol or symbols next to each entry.

Your goal is to transform all the negative characteristics into positive ones. You can accomplish this by breathing the element that you wish to work with into your body through your pores, concentrating on the specific aspects of the element associated with the characteristic you wish to build or to remove. When you work with an element in this way, it is vital to stay very clear about which aspect of the element you take in.

For example, you might think of yourself as lazy, which indicates a lack of Fire. When you work with Fire, it is the energizing properties of Fire that you are calling on. If you were working on issues around being timid or fearful, you would also call on the element Fire; however, you would be asking for the courageous properties, another very different aspect of Fire.

Or let's suppose you are flighty and ungrounded, or can't seem to get any consistency in your day-to-day activities. This problem would call for working with the element of Earth to create more structure and stability in your life.

You can also change your temperature working in this way, using Water as a cooling agent and Fire to warm yourself. Tibetan masters have a highly developed relationship with the elements, as evidenced in their ability to change their temperatures in harsh conditions.

When you first practice this technique, work in only one direction at a time—put all your attention toward inviting the aspects of a particular element into yourself. After you get comfortable with the process, you will be able to take in one aspect of an element and remove one during a single process. You will be using the entire organ of pores in order to facilitate filling your body with the element, rather than focusing on any specific part.

EXERCISE

Sample Elemental Transformation

I suggest you read these sample instructions, which focus on working with Fire to remedy laziness, then adapt the instructions to fit the character quality you wish to work on.

Start with one of the qualities of your character that you've listed in the negative column. Let's suppose you have written *lazy;* perhaps you simply can't get enough energy together to function as you would like. This problem would call for working with the element of Fire. Close your eyes and imagine yourself sitting inside a red, downward-pointed triangle or pyramid. See yourself as an empty vessel, your outer edges shimmering. Focus on that outer shell surface, your pores, and find their rhythm. It is usually very fast. As you cannot sustain breathing at that speed, synchronize your breathing to find a resonance between your breath and the rhythm of your pores. . . .

Once in resonance, slow down your breathing to a comfortable rate, and begin to envision yourself inhaling deeply the element of Fire, or more specifically, that aspect of Fire that is most stimulating, into your body through your pores. Because you are using your entire shell as the doorway, it will only take a few breaths to fill yourself completely. You might find yourself getting quite warm as you take in Fire in this way. . . .

When you are entirely filled with this Fire, breathe slowly, holding the stimulating energy of Fire in your body as you focus on what it will be like in the future when this aspect of the Fire element has become part of your being. Take a moment to picture a time when your body and mind respond to your energetic needs from that place of abundant Fire; know the vitality that this Fire element will leave with you. . . .

When you have seen and felt the difference, and know it for your future, you can begin to release the Fire element with each exhale. It is very important to get every last spark of Fire out of your body, exhaling through your pores.

No matter which element you are working with, it is necessary to release *all* of the element when you exhale it. Remember, this is an alchemical process in which the power remains after the element has been removed.

When you have mastered this technique, you can begin to work the elements in both directions as you continue your practice. For example, on your list you could have a need for some aspect of Earth at the same time that you recognize an area where you have too much Earth. You might have a situation in which you need more structure or order, and yet there are areas in your character where you perceive that you are rigid and inflexible. As you inhale the structure and order of Earth, stay focused on that aspect. After you have transformed that energy into its most positive result in your body and just before you exhale, begin to focus on that aspect of Earth that you want to remove, and see yourself responding to life from that less rigid, more flexible place. Then, as you exhale, use your intention to release your rigidity with the Earth element as it leaves your body through your pores. It is okay to repeat the process with an element and deal with additional aspects as needed.

If you work on at least one elemental transformation each day, you will find results in a short time. I also use this method to deal with situations as they arise, when I notice that I require the addition of an element, or to reduce an element in my system.

PART IV

COMPLETION— ALCHEMICAL GOLD

19
THE FOUR PRINCIPLES OF ALCHEMICAL HEALING

THERE ARE FOUR PRINCIPLE ELEMENTS that are integral to the structure of any Alchemical Healing. To illustrate the interdependence of these elements, I will use the image of an arch.

In an arch, each brick is an integral part whose absence would weaken the whole of the structure. The four Alchemical Healing principles illustrated by the arch include one's personal skill, assistance based on relationships in the spirit realms, divine intervention, and gratitude.

PERSONAL SKILL

Personal skill includes the abilities and techniques you develop through practicing the exercises in this book. These provide the basis for any healing in which you participate. As you practice the exercises, you hone your edge and advance your skill level. Personal skill also includes any additional healing practices you have learned

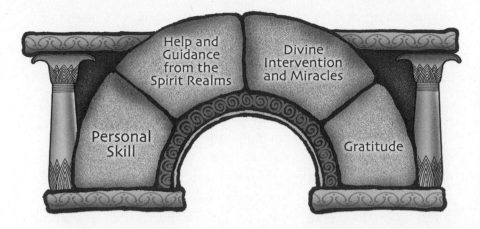

Figure 19.1. *The Four Principles of Alchemical Healing*

from all other systems and traditions you have worked with. Discrimination and communication skills, your ability to set your intention, to focus, and to give love also contribute to this portion of the arch, as do music skills and any other gifts you have developed that you bring to the work. Skill is your ability to make use of your talents and put your knowledge into practice. The more you practice, the more you will expand, strengthen, and adapt whatever skills you have to the situation.

HELP AND GUIDANCE FROM THE SPIRIT REALMS

Here is where the relationships you have made with the elements, totems, and other spirit guides are integrated into your practice. This principle brings balance to your personal skills and widens the scope of your perspective. Without this section of the arch, you significantly limit your possibilities. Your skills are also appreciated here, as they afford you the opportunity to co-create with the allies, and you reap the inspiration and rewards that come with teamwork.

It is important to distinguish when and to whom it is appropriate to call. Remember to stay present to new possibilities and notice any new entity that shows up to help. Your ability to recognize and invoke allies is a skill; the contributions of the allies themselves constitute the second principle.

DIVINE INTERVENTION

This is the segment of the healing work where you know you have done everything that you can, and you ask for help. Then get out of the way, with full knowledge that the actual energy being utilized is coming from the unfathomable Mystery.

Miracles do happen. Another way of describing miracles is divine intervention. Components that are beyond our comprehension enter into every healing ritual. These include intuition, coincidence, and gifts from the universe that you did not anticipate and could not have expected. They provide inspiration, transformation, and the Mystery. It is imperative to allow space in every healing for this principle, which requires faith in the process. This principle is undermined by expectation for specific outcomes and by filling the space constantly with doing.

GRATITUDE

The principle of gratitude includes the honoring of the entire magical structure as well as any individual entities or elements involved. You may offer gratitude at any time during the process, and always at the end before disconnecting from the person or situation on which you are working. The process of gratitude continues as the lessons of the healing are slowly understood and integrated. Illness is a great teacher, one that requires respect and gratitude if it is to reveal its deepest teachings.

The importance of gratitude cannot be overstated. As young children we are taught to give thanks to all who show us kindness. It is a fundamental principle of etiquette, and a "good" upbringing teaches us the importance of saying "thank you." As we grow and mature, this simple lesson becomes so much a part of who we are that it becomes easy to take the obvious for granted. The profound depths of the meaning of gratitude can be lost to shallow lip service.

Sharing your gifts is a form of gratitude in action. Gratitude is the food and nourishment that we give back to spirit, and its most potent form is attention.

★ ☽ ★

If any of the above principles are missing, the structure of the arch, although it might not come crashing down, will be weakened. For the sustained power of any healing, all four must be present and appropriately honored.

When I was diagnosed with breast cancer in December of 1991, I thought I could continue my life as it was. My book, *The Golden Cauldron*, had just been published, and I was preparing to go on the road to publicize my greatest achievement. I even had the audacity to consult my calendar to see just when I would have time to deal with the pesky lump I had discovered.

Attempts to continue living life in the fast lane came to an abrupt halt following two surgeries and the advent of the intensive chemotherapy protocol that was recommended. I found myself flat on my back and with no recourse but to surrender to my fate.

In the new and unexpected direction of my journey, I chose to combine the tools of my healing work with those of traditional Western medicine. My intention to fight for my life and use all the skill that was available to me, both mine and others, comprised the first fundamental section of the arch. There were days when I could do no more than pay attention to my breath for a few moments, and other days when I was able to devote strong attention to my healing; sometimes it was enough to simply lay my hands on different parts of my body with the intention to let the energy flow, and at other times I could delve more deeply into my medicine bag of tricks. The key point is to remember to use the skills you have developed.

The second principle was also in effect every step of the way. My urgent call for help went out immediately, and the guides that responded stayed with me throughout, giving graciously of their support and guidance. Looking back, it is the presence of the guides and allies that stand out more than the pain, discomfort, and misery of the initiation by poisoning that was the bitter medicine of my struggle.

Although there were numerous moments of divine intervention during my cancer treatment, a special epiphany of particular grace occurred one day as I was lying in the hammock in our garden. It was springtime and the sun warming the land brought out the insects and birds—I remember hearing the buzzing of bees. Our three ducks waddled up from the pond, quacking as they came toward me. These simple duck sounds became trumpets that heralded a shift in my awareness, and I suddenly knew that all of the spirits of the nature that surrounded me were conspiring to bring me back to health. In a glorious moment of presence, I knew myself as an integral part of the fabric of creation, and I knew that I would live.

The hand of God, Creator, the Mystery, Great Spirit, Allah, or whatever name you use—the Divine is evident in the epiphanies that magically arise during any extended healing journey, and that provide both the clues and the treasures as the hunt for life's meaning continues. Even if the eventual result is death, as it ultimately is for us all, the process itself is a sacred journey. The magical moments along the way are impossible to create, or even imagine; yet the mere act of conscious intention and action serve as invitations or invocations for spirit.

Regardless of the misery, the pain, the sorrow, remembrance of thanksgiving creates a soothing balm for the soul. When we are suffering and confused, there is great solace in counting our blessings, finding, even in the darkest and most despairing times, that voice of gratitude that brings a shaft of light upon which our spirits can rise.

When we are practicing Alchemical Healing, or any other practice, art, or function of life that attracts the gifts of spirit, it is our gratitude that expresses our acknowledgment and honoring of the source of these gifts. Without these, our tasks in life would be so much more bland and difficult.

OFFERINGS

Remembering to say thank you is an expression of gratitude that is always welcome. The sense of gratitude can be run through you in much the same way as the Universal Life Force, according to your intention. It *feels* wonderful to be engaged in the act of honoring through gratitude, and it strengthens the connection with the unseen forces.

When working ceremonially, creating ritual, and doing healing work, there are times and situations that call for more. For example, you learned in Chapter 11 about how important it is to offer energy to the family of the plant allies that come to assist you. Following are some suggestions for offerings that you can apply to different situations as they come up. The simple prayer ceremony that I suggest is one that always includes gratitude as one of its main ingredients.

CEREMONY OF THANKS

My early teacher, Oh Shinnah, taught me to keep a small altar that includes cornmeal, tobacco, and an abalone shell or other receptacle, and sage, cedar, or whatever incense is available. Upon rising in the morning, smudge yourself, then take a pinch of tobacco and offer it to the six directions. (Some people like to include a seventh, so that it is East, South, West, North, Above, Below, Within.) Put your gratitude and your heartfelt prayers into the tobacco. Then scatter the pinch onto the earth, weather and other circumstances permitting. In the evening, do the same thing using the cornmeal instead of tobacco. Keep a small receptacle, a shell or bowl, in which you can place your tobacco and cornmeal offerings if the weather is inclement or if for any reason you cannot go outside. These you can take out and offer to the earth, a plant, or a tree later, when convenient. Be sure to remember to give thanks for all the blessings and lessons of your life, and for those around you that you love, and for the sustenance that maintains you.

The most common traditional "offering plants" in the Americas are tobacco and cornmeal. Tobacco has a more masculine feel to it, and cornmeal is decidedly feminine, associated with the great corn mother of the Hopi and other western Native traditions. I use them interchangeably, according to what I have available to me; however, I was initially taught to offer tobacco for my morning prayers and cornmeal in the evening.

Throughout the Americas, tobacco is a sacred plant, said to be the favored food for the spirits and allies of shamans. I often use tobacco as my offering for various ceremonies. It seems to hold prayers and gratitude in a way that when the spirits are called, they can tell what's in the heart of the person who is praying by the thoughts that are held in the tobacco offering.

When I travel to Egypt or other foreign soil, or even other places in my own country, I always make an offering to the spirits of the land, asking permission to be there and offering gratitude for my safe arrival and the possibilities to come. Until I have engaged in this simple ritual, I may find myself not quite connected to my new surroundings.

Water is precious and sacred. Although we cannot live without it, we tend to take it for granted. It is beneficial to remember the value of water in our lives, and to give thanks for water much as we give thanks for the foods we eat. It can be a powerful discipline to occasionally give up water for a period of time to remind ourselves of the sacredness of water. Muslims fast without food or water during the days of Ramadan, as do Jews for Yom Kippur. (Keep in mind that children and the infirm are exempted.) Please use common sense regarding your physical well-being before you engage in a fast that includes not drinking water.

Saying grace over the food before a meal is common practice in many traditions. Some Native American tribes create a "spirit plate" at every meal, offering a tiny portion of each food served with prayers of thanksgiving for the nurturing and sustenance we receive from our meals. The spirit plate is left out for the spirits to receive the nourishment of our gratitude, and, one way or another, the food almost always disappears.

GATHERING PLANTS AND HERBS

Oh Shinnah was the first teacher to share the art of offering with me. It was 1973, and the siege of Wounded Knee was happening. I was living in Mill Valley, California, when she took me with her to gather certain herbs to be used as medicine for the Natives stranded on the reservation in South Dakota. She taught me that when *wild crafting,* it is important to never take all of what is available at any stand where the herbs are growing. Find the "Grandmother" plant, the largest or oldest plant in the stand, and offer tobacco to the six directions in honor of the plant and what you plan to do with it. Tell the plant your need, and request permission to take what you require. Then go to smaller plants in the area and take a little from each one until you have what you need. Give thanks to the Grandmother and to each plant from which you harvest. While harvesting, take your time and allow the plant to let you know which parts are ready to be taken. Remember that to overharvest not only deprives other people of whatever medicine you are gathering, but it depletes the resource and may endanger the plant family's survival in that location.

FRAGRANCE OFFERINGS

Incenses of all sorts were used in ancient times to purge spirits and cleanse spaces. Sweet resins from frankincense and myrrh trees were highly valued in the Middle and Far East, carried by caravans over vast distances to find their way as exotic relief for the stench of the cities of Europe and Asia. From images on the carved walls of the temples of ancient Egypt to the contemporary cathedrals where smoking censers are carried throughout to purify the space, incense is seen as a fundamental part of ritual.

Sage is, in our region, the most common smudge for cleansing a space. There are many species of salvia that when burned create a pungent odor. Mugwort can be substituted, and is also used to conjure dreams. Cedars and junipers are employed as well, and their fragrant smoke purifies the body, while the sweet grasses of the plains are braided and burned to spread a fragrance similar to vanilla, which is used to call in beneficial spirits. In Mexico and South America, it is the resin of copal that has been used in ritual throughout time. Indigenous shamans the world over had their means of altering the ambient fragrance of space in order to banish unwanted spirits and invite allies.

Whenever you light any incense, you have an opportunity to extend gratitude, both to the plant spirits you are working with, and as an honoring of the alchemical process of transformation in which you are engaged.

THE GIVEAWAY

An important expression of gratitude for many Native American tribes, and other cultures as well, is the *giveaway*. After a vision, a healing, a battle won, or any rite of passage, gifting is appropriate, and in many cultures, expected. In some tribes, the wealth of people is measured not by what they have, but by what they give away. Imagine a world in which this was the standard.

Charity and tithing are important aspects of religious and cultural mores the world over as forms of spiritual offering that honor the commitment of devotees to their beliefs.

Regardless of one's motivation, giving stimulates the movement of energy, and spirit responds. Pay special attention when you intuit that it is time to pass on a special "treasure." Sacred implements, such as feathers, rattles, crystals, and other meaningful items, will tell you when they want to move on, and to whom they should be given. When you give freely, whether it is money or food or Alchemical Healing, you are rewarded in unexpected ways. Giving away is a vital part of the magic.

ATTENTION

And finally, *attention* is the deepest form of gratitude, and whether it is to your family, your friends, or your spirit allies, the attention you offer results in deeper, more meaningful relationships; and relationships are what truly matter.

20
THE WISDOM
OF THE HEART

ALTHOUGH ALCHEMICAL HEALING IS ostensibly a collection of healing tools, for the serious student it can be a way of life, a path that can lead to spiritual awakening and, ultimately, enlightenment. As this path continues to unfold, certain discoveries are inevitable. One of the most important of these is the ability and necessity to perceive the world from the heart. For many of us this requires an alteration of the way we have previously moved through life.

No longer can we listen only with our head, or run our lives from our will, our sexual desires, or our emotions. When we are totally present, we are listening with the heart. In ancient Egypt when bodies were mummified the brains were sucked out and discarded, while the heart was saved, put in a special vase, and venerated as the seat of intelligence.

When we perceive events through our hearts, we don't have issues that constrict us such as anger or revenge. Although we may experience sorrow or concern, our love and compassion for the human condition and our desire for people to be the best that they can be will sway our opinions and our responses. When we are fully in our hearts, we have no judgments—the usual polarities that dominate the old paradigm, such as good/bad and right/wrong, are absent.

If you walk past any playground where children are playing together, you are likely to hear the sound of laughter and see some children joyfully cooperating with one another. There might also be a bully in the group, and perhaps some kids are sitting alone, sad. When you are coming from your heart, you don't feel the need to judge—this is good, this is bad. You just simply embrace the whole playground and every child in it; you perceive the perfection and wish for each child a full and wonderful life. It's a matter of going from judging every activity to appreciating every activity.

Although we may thrive on the love that is directed to us from others, we are ultimately responsible for the tending of our own heart flame, and it is important to keep that fire kindled and radiant. The more we focus on our heart center, the more we are able to stay centered within it.

When I forget or lose my heart-centered focus, I tend to fall back into old patterns of behavior, especially in my responses to curves and unexpected changes. It is then easy for me to become constricted and judgmental, and to worry and make up scenarios based on assumptions. The concern I create can turn to fear or anger, the need to manipulate, or some other undesirable reaction. Before I know it my mind, emotions, or will has once again taken over. Following are some examples of a few of the personality traits you may recognize that are associated with the various chakra centers, especially when the heart center is bypassed.

A person coming primarily from the first chakra is often motivated by issues of survival or security. When choices and decisions are made with those issues at the fore, the result would likely be greed or hoarding—an insecurity about ever having enough. And when one determines a course of action based mainly on their personal security, chances are he or she may become fearful, even cowardly.

When people make choices based on sexual desire or emotional charge, they are usually dwelling in their second chakra. We are all familiar with reactions based on emotions such as lust or self-pity.

Such actions inevitably create more problems than solutions, and keep us out of our center, and out of our hearts.

When coming from Will, our attention is centered in our ego, in our personal power as expressed through the third chakra. When we direct our actions from this center we tend to be passionate and creative about what we are doing, and often accomplish our goals by force of will. I was very good at this way of surviving, and always felt justified because I knew myself to be right and powerful, and politically correct. Often I could make things happen in spite of overwhelming odds, and I was convinced that my survival depended on this ability. It is hard for many of us to change an ingrained habit pattern like this because it requires giving up a level of control that we are sure is vital. When people are acting from their will, they may find themselves dictating to others, self-righteous in their assessments, impatient and manipulative, insecure, and quick to criticize.

People coming from Mind are focused at the fifth chakra, a place of reason and intellect where, without sufficient awareness in the heart, they might find themselves rationalizing and spinning stories in their head, perfectly logical from their point of view. They might also be invested in communicating their personal perspective, convinced that they are right, and sure that others are simply not getting it. Moving from Mind to Heart requires loosening our grip on our sense of certainty. I was always able to calculate with my mind as though I was playing a game of chess, looking forward as far as possible beyond the next move. I would then proceed from my will—my determination and desire strong and right, and my course of action appropriate and defendable. Yet sometimes my decision making was an exercise in rationalization. Perhaps the reasons behind my decisions were more self-serving than I cared to admit. Reason is useful, and it provides a stable base for making appropriate choices; however, if we allow pure heartfelt inspiration, we often discover something new and unexpected that we could not find through reason alone.

The higher chakras, sixth and above, must be approached with utmost respect. These are doorways to higher consciousness and the universal mind. The avatars, shamans, and others who pursue spiritual enlightenment in these domains undergo rigorous training and discipline. Those who explore and dwell in these infinite dimensions without being grounded and balanced in the lower centers, especially the heart, risk delusion and insanity. Because this tendency was borne out quite graphically during the explorations of my youth, it has been a primary objective for me to find and offer safe pathways to awakened states of being. In my ongoing search for the healing and transformation that results in spiritual growth, I have concluded that the heart is our true center of being. It is our heart that is weighed against the feather of Maät, the Egyptian goddess of balance, order, and truth. When we come from the perspective of the heart, we are connected to an inherent intelligence that serves our highest good.

Although I still struggle with sustaining heart-centered awareness, I am now able to see the change in my point of reference, and the quality of my life has improved markedly. Whereas I could not have envisioned my current state of consciousness from the old paradigm, I can now recognize when I have drifted off center and am no longer making decisions from a place of clarity. I tend now to move more slowly, yet go farther faster. The vicious cycle of having to be right, or of thinking I am creating the whole show, can be broken with a return to center, and to a strong and healthy heart flame, in the light of which I am able to make heartfelt choices based in compassion and love.

Following is an empowerment that helps you return to and remain in your heart center. It is a rewiring of the energetic circuits that elevate your center of power and wisdom through a movement from Will to Heart—from ego to essence. It is about the distinction between what serves us personally, and what we serve—between our personal will and Divinity.

This attunement helps you to perceive the world from the heart chakra. Sustaining that point of perception is a constant work in progress. Initially you have to work harder to return to the heart; it takes ingenuity to overcome old habits. As C. S. Lewis expresses it: "I insisted that God ought to appear in the temple I had built for him, not knowing that he cares only for temples building and not at all for temples built."*

After you've brought yourself back to the heart so often that your body remembers, when it becomes habit, then you will default to the heart whenever you fully relax, or when you achieve a place of absolute serenity. The opportunity is inherent in the process. With a shift in your attention, you will be able to return to center anytime you get thrown off. When you relax and surrender completely you will be back, totally present, held in the soft caress of the compassionate heart—connected to everything and everyone, with respect and admiration for every living being. There is comfort in being part of the larger tribe of life rather than an isolated individual.

Once you have taken the following journey, there will be a noticeable shift when you project from the heart with your breath. Continuing the Heart Breath as a practice will help keep your heart flame strong and help you to relax and perceive your life, no matter the chaos of any particular situation, from a place of love and compassion. This initiation is meant to be taken only once, and only by those who have familiarized themselves with and practiced with the element Akasha. The elements of the empowerment will become embedded in your energetic systems through your heart center, and will remain so throughout this life. In the beginning of the journey, you will be asked to breathe Akasha into your heart on the Heart Breath. This instruction is for this journey *only*, to prepare the heart for the emanation that will be given. It is important to be seated, as, even though you should have become accustomed to working with Akasha by the time you take this journey, you are likely to get drowsy.

A *sigil* is a magical symbol encoded with the energy of one's personal vibrational signature. It radiates a power that is unique to the individual for whom it was designed. Your sigil, upon which you can meditate for deeper understanding of self, will be conferred during the empowerment. It will continue to radiate and amplify

*C. S. Lewis, *Surprised by Joy* (New York: Harcourt Brace Jovanovich, 1955), 167.

your vibrational signature, especially when you are engaged in working from the heart. Your sigil also increases your receptivity to others who are emanating from their hearts.

Avalokitesvara is the Tibetan embodiment of compassion. When I was in Tibet I was privileged to go to the ancient monastery at Samye, perhaps the oldest in Tibet, where there is a chapel devoted to him. A huge statue of Avalokitesvara fills the chapel. It radiates a thousand arms, each with an eye in the palm, symbolizing the all-seeing hands that reach out to those in distress. Just as Thoth can shapeshift into any form in order to express wisdom, so Avalokitesvara is said to be able to enter all forms in order to relieve suffering. All of the archetypes and deities of compassion are said to be related to this ancient being. He emanates the same energy as Kuan Yin in the Orient, Chenrezig in Tibet, Mary to Christians, Isis and Sekhet to ancient Egyptians, White Buffalo Calf woman to Native Americans, and many, many more. During the journey that follows, the ray of compassion that is appropriate for you—whether a deity, a totem, or an archetype—will be birthed in your heart flame, and activated by Avalokitesvara.

The emanation that comes to you in this journey will be awakened whenever you practice the Heart Breath, and whenever you focus on your heart center and rekindle your heart flame. The power intrinsic to this being will be added to whatever and wherever you send your healing intentions and energies.

INITIATION

FROM WILL TO HEART

Set up your sacred space and prepare for this journey by smudging and calling the directions. . . .

Close your eyes, ground and center. . . .

Find the eternal flame that dwells in your heart center. Feed

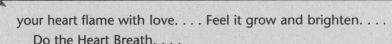

your heart flame with love. . . . Feel it grow and brighten. . . .

Do the Heart Breath. . . .

Invoke Akasha by drawing the Akashic egg symbol above your head, and breathe Akasha into your body to fill your heart with Akasha. It will automatically convert any negative emotions there, and release them as you exhale. Because you are using Akasha, they will dissolve back into the Akashic realm. . . .

In your heart center, you begin to make out the presence of a lotus flower bud growing within your heart flame. It is closed at first, and as you continue to breathe the Heart Breath it begins to open, petal by petal. . . .

Pull another round of Akasha, this time from your hands into and around you. The influx of Akasha fills you, inside and out, and obscures your vision and sensitivities for a moment. When it clears, you are sitting at a long and narrow white table. You cannot recognize the people who are sitting on either side or across from you, but you are aware that this table extends to infinity in both directions, and you are all waiting. . . .

You hear the shuffle of a deck of cards, and the snick as someone you can't see turns a card face up in front of you. You will not be able to perceive the features on the card at this time.

Keep breathing. . . . Continue to stare at the card. Breathe slowly and deeply. During the next exhale, a hand reaches into your third chakra, into your solar plexus, and draws a fine thread of aka from within your third center, pulls it out and up, and carefully places it into your heart center, right into the center of the opening lotus. . . .

As you continue gazing at your card, the focus becomes a little sharper, but you are still having difficulty making out the details. Continue breathing the Heart Breath. On the next exhale, you are aware of a hand reaching into your second chakra. It enters and gathers a fine filament from your second chakra, carefully withdraws it, and gently attaches that to the center of the opening lotus in the fire of your heart. . . .

Notice that certain symbols on the card are becoming more meaningful and are beginning to make sense. You might notice a feeling of hope and intuition. There is recognition that this is your card. There is none other like it. This is your sigil. . . .

By the time the connection between your second, third, and heart chakras is complete, the lotus blossom is fully opened and emitting a luscious fragrance. As the symbol on your card comes into clarity, you feel the blessing of the essence of compassion enter your heart. . . .

An archetype of compassion rises from the core of the lotus and appears in your heart flame. This being can be a deity or totem or any emanation of compassion that has come to join you, someone full of love and warmth, whose mere presence overwhelms anything but your love and compassion for yourself and all others. Feel this being as it awakens inside you. Welcome it and allow it to manifest in as much detail as possible. . . .

Now pick up your card and take a moment to study the features of you sigil. . . . Hold it close to your chest. Feel it dissolve into your heart. The final, complete symbol is deeply encoded in your memory. It grounds the connection that has been made, and resonates with all your chakras, providing a direct link between each of your chakras and your heart. The symbol on the card is a sacred, living sigil and will continue to radiate from your heart flame as your personal identity signature.

The emanation of compassion will stay and work with you and help you to sustain the transition from your will to your heart. It is an intrinsic part of the flame, and once embedded, is connected to your entire chakra system.

Be sure to express your gratitude to all the elements that came together during this journey. . . .

Ground and center yourself, and sit quietly for a few moments before opening your eyes. . . .

ALCHEMICAL TONGLEN

The archetypal being that came to you and the sigil that is your magical vibratory signature will always be there. You can remember your sigil at any time and meditate on the symbol with great benefit. You can connect with the indwelling emanation of compassion simply by focusing your attention on your heart flame. It will express itself into whatever you are trying to accomplish. It is of value to be aware of and consciously engage this emanation when you do the practices that follow.

There is an age-old Tibetan practice called *Tonglen* that develops compassion. The literal meaning for the word *Tonglen* is giving and receiving. In Tibetan, *tong* means to give, and *len* to receive. There will come a time, if you practice regularly and become mindful of your breath in an integrated way, when you will find yourself comfortable with a more Tonglen-like approach to healing. With Tonglen one uses the Heart Breath to literally transform an emotionally toxic environment. Tonglen can be practiced for self-healing or for relieving pain and emotional angst for others, and can be extended beyond individuals to include all who may be suffering in similar ways.

In Alchemical Healing, this is done simply by doing the Heart Breath with awareness that you are transforming the disharmonious energies around you in the crucible of your heart flame. To do this practice effectively, you must first work with the Heart Breath on yourself, clearing your own inner space and body.* It is helpful to acknowledge the compassionate being that now lives within your heart. After you have accomplished that, you can allow discord, or pain, or any form of suffering to enter your body from external sources as you inhale. It is vital to distinguish between what is yours and what is grist for this alchemical mill. Do not retain the toxins! Keep your focus on your heart, and allow

---

*Note: Giraffe, as totem animal, and the Giraffe Journey, "Seeing from the Heart," from *Power Animal Meditations* (Rochester, Vt.: Bear & Co., 2001) is beneficial for sustaining heart-centered awareness.

yourself to perceive consciously as the transformation occurs in your heart flame; then send the purified energies back out into the world through your heart center.

In Alchemical Healing mastering the invigorating Heart Breath and completing the "From Will to Heart" empowerment are prerequisites to being able to transform toxic energies and emotions from our surroundings into love.

Please do not practice this technique with radiation sickness or radiation therapy, or with the intention of transforming radiation that has been released into the environment. I tried it once and became very ill.

COMPASSIONATE LISTENING

As you integrate the practices that have brought you thus far, you may want to try a more advanced practice such as the one following—another Alchemical Healing version of Tonglen. This practice allows one to experience another's point of view, a useful tool in remembering that we are all one, and that adverse points of view can be understood best from a place of resonance, where we comprehend and own them.

To live harmoniously in the midst of diversity, each of us must confront the differences between ourselves and others whose values and beliefs are unlike our own. To do this fully, we must be willing to give up our preconceptions. This requires a practice of attentive and compassionate listening, without expectation or judgment—a practice that would give us a new perspective, a different life experience, regardless of what is happening around us.

Compassion is not just about feeling sorry for someone or something; it is also about being fully present with whatever is happening. During this practice you might experience the emotions of the person you are perceiving, yet there is an honoring as you observe and learn. Although you don't *take on* the other's personal experience as your own, you do recognize the depth and similarity of certain fundamental aches we all share.

Being compassionate leads to right action. Very different results come from acting out of compassion rather than acting out of conflict or guilt, hate or revenge. In Alchemical Healing this practice is called Becoming Another, or Compassionate Listening. The ultimate goal of this work is to recognize how we are the same at our core, regardless of our outward differences. Perhaps the most important benefit is to be able to receive, to feel, and to know another's belief system, no matter how alien it appears from our own. The key, of course, is to receive this information without judgments. That's the hard part; yet if we can do it, we can learn to love and respect one another.

You need to be prepared for the possibility that when practicing Becoming Another, you might merge with the person you are observing. Although many of us have forgotten, we are all interconnected. Until we are 100 percent at that place of loving another as ourselves, we can continue to fall prey to divisive emotions.

Another compensation for this work is that if you do this practice, not just comprehend it but do it, you will develop the ability to communicate with others no matter where they are in the world. In the modern age of communications, technologies like telephones and computer e-mail are great conveniences. We need to remember, however, that in relying on them we are trading our ability to communicate in the inherent ways of our ancestors. We can remember our telepathic potential through this work; yet that too is only a small part of the benefit of this practice.

This is not a practice to be taken lightly. It requires considerable focus and concentration. I recommend you start with a person in your life with whom you have some disagreement but who does not feel threatening to you before you tackle those whom you perceive as greater adversaries.

It is possible that when you synchronize your breath with the person according to the instructions below, you may feel a merging take place, so proceed slowly and carefully, approaching this as a sacred ritual, and with clear intention. Be sure not to lose yourself in the process. You will be involved in observation, and you must remain in a state of compassion and love. Although it is not necessary, you can invite a totem or allies to be with you to witness, protect, and support you. It is important that you enter this process with integrity—you are not there to change anything, only to be compassionate in the moment—and to listen. There is tremendous potential for creating love through this work. Take courage in your underlying desire to know truth.

MEDITATION

Compassionate Listening/Becoming Another

Sit in a place of comfort where there will be no distractions. You may wish to smudge the space or light incense and a candle. Allow yourself the time between each instruction to see, feel, and know with as many senses as you can bring to your focus.

Choose the person you wish to understand. Close your eyes. Ground and center yourself. . . .

Focus on your heart. Find the eternal flame that lives within your heart center, and feed that flame with love. . . . The flame will brighten, allowing your heart to open to whatever happens, without expectation or judgment. . . .

Picture the person you want to understand in front of you. Observe this person. Watch them. See all the details, or, if you don't see in pictures, feel or sense or know. . . . Notice how this person breathes. What is the rhythm of his or her breath? Pay close attention to the nuances of the breathing, and begin to breathe with the person. . . . Synchronize your breathing. . . . If the other person's breath is too fast or too slow for your physical comfort, then just imagine yourself synchronizing your breathing. . . .

As you continue to breathe together, you will begin to notice thoughts (perhaps in images or words, or through whatever senses are engaged) that just come up and enter your consciousness. Let these thoughts enter without placing any judgments on them. Pay close attention. . . .

Submerge into your own psyche and seek the bridge between you and the other person . . . Regardless of what thoughts or images you perceive, remain neutral and allow love and compassion to flow from you into the person you are linked to in this way. Stay with this for a while. . . .

When you feel complete with this experience, disengage your attention from the person you have been observing. Bring your attention back into yourself and your heart flame. Pour love upon your heart flame and feel the warmth and radiance flow through your entire being. . . .

Ground and center yourself. . . .

It is important that when you connect to a person in this way that you respectfully disconnect when you are finished with the exercise.

May the power of love and compassion transform our fear, our hatred, and our confusion into creative energy that can be used to heal and to nurture *all our relations*.

LOVE AS AN ELEMENT

From the first to the fourth chakras, we are working with energies associated with the earth, energies that are dependent on the laws of gravity and physics. The heart center is the nexus point between the earth and what is beyond the laws of physics and gravity. It's like a platform, or a point of departure. The heart is associated with the present moment and connected to everything at the same time.

In this system, there is no specific element that is associated with the heart center. If I were to name another element for this place, it would be love.

It occurs to me that in all the discussions about the elements and other allies that help with the Alchemical Healing work, the most present and yet most elusive to articulation has been love. Yet love is the motivation, the medium, the expression, and the container for all healing. Love connects us all and is the force that joins us together with joy. Love permeates our known reality, binding the disparate parts of our larger selves. It is the quintessential healing component. In an environment where love is cultivated, less healing is needed. Although it is not considered an element by any traditions of which I am aware, by its fundamental and essential nature, it could most certainly be included as one.

I learned a wonderful process from a shaman friend who is also a psychologist, Reuben Wolff. I was privileged to witness as Reuben, in one session, held space for Mark to shed issues that had plagued him from infancy. It is beyond the scope of my articulation in psychology to describe the content and mechanics of his method, but I can attest to the results, and report what I saw. Reuben is a master at embodying love, directing it, and holding his strength and presence without wavering, for however long it takes for the fear or pain in someone to lessen. His skill lies in his ability to engender trust in whomever he is working with—trust is the key. It is unfortunate that in our culture so often in the presence of pure love, one's first thoughts might be "What is this person after? What does he want?"

My experience with Reuben's work caused me to reflect on the action of love in Alchemical Healing. Love is a constant—all energies generated in this work are embued with love, more or less consciously. Do we take love for granted in healing? Perhaps by naming it, by actively calling on it and honoring its presence, both the healer and the one who is being healed will become more mindful and allow more love into their processes and their lives. As a healer, it is important to cultivate and express love in all your actions.

HOLDING PRACTICE

I have adapted what I experienced with Reuben into the following technique for Alchemical Healing. Because it requires physical contact, it is vital to have established a solid relationship before you begin and to receive permission from the person you're working with. This relationship should be built on trust and impeccability. It is the trust that allows the person to relax in the knowledge that she is and will be safe, so that she can open fully, and receive the love that is offered. It is the love imbued with the quality of strength that holds the container. I have used this technique with people who are in acute chronic pain, such as with fibromyalgia, and for people who are living with extreme stress and tension. Once you begin, try to hold your position for at least ten minutes. The process is better served the longer you can maintain it—try an hour if you can.

The technique is to simply hold and support the person. Maintain absolute integrity and create a trustworthy container in which the person you are working with feels bathed in love. He must be so lovingly held as to allow him to enter what is perhaps the scariest core of his being. While held in this way, one might remember the first time a defensive pattern was created, perhaps even during precognitive infancy. If emotions are released, it is imperative to continue holding until resolution is achieved. Perhaps she will be comfortable enough to remember the first time that she perceived, and consequently held as truth that maybe there was something wrong with her, something unlovable. The subtle undercurrent of fear created by such a deeply ingrained pattern results in a rigidity of being that is often not recognized until it is gone. Core behaviors such as this one dictate the endless games that, although they are fundamental constructs that we perceive as essential for our survival, must be released in order to access a state of presence. Remember, these "constructs" were perfect for the moment when they were created, although at present they no longer serve you and may even be detrimental. In order to identify such core issues there must be confidence in the absolute safety of the process. That net of safety for this work is the nurturing benevolence of unconditional love.

Once a core issue is identified, you can then conduct the transformational process to remove all vestiges of the offending pattern.

(See the advanced techniques presented in this book.) Just being held in this way, however, will give tremendous benefit. And you must remain consistently vigilant about always giving the power to the person you're working with so that it is they, with conscious choice, that determine whether and when to move forward.

Example

I have a friend whose health complaints and symptoms have become debilitating as the vicious cycle of pain, medication, and more pain have taken their toll. I offered her a session in which I hoped to reduce her immediate symptoms and give her some tools to help her in her ongoing struggle. Yet when the time came, I could see that she was about to break from the tension of holding herself rigid to ward off one thing and another.

I got comfortable on my couch, with good back support, then asked her to turn around so I could reach around her and she could rest against me. Then I suggested she relax and guided her muscle by muscle, until she finally was able to relinquish her body tension. I then simply held her and rocked her slightly. I noticed that even when she seemed as though she was in full repose, there was always another level of relaxation to attain.

The concept of being held was so foreign to her that the results were dramatic. Within about five minutes, the pain that had been wracking her body almost totally disappeared. I just kept holding her, reminding her that she needn't do anything but relax and breathe, and that she was totally deserving of love. So simple, yet so profound.

In order to help her to sustain the results we had obtained, I introduced her to my Bear totem ally. When she was able to perceive the bear, I pointed out to her how the bear would hold her in the same way as I had, and that whenever she felt the tension return, she could rest in the powerful, massive, and strong body of Bear and be held and supported.

Isis, the Egyptian goddess who graces the cover of this book, can also be invoked to hold and embrace the person. She will gather a person into her wings, which often makes the person feel as though he or she has come home.

Alchemical Healing techniques do not often require connecting in the way of physical touch; however, sometimes there is no substitute for pure, unconditional love and support for the body. If holding is inappropriate, put the power of your intention into a very large hug and find an opportunity to share it that way.

Alchemical Healing is inclusive of all tools and dimensions that are available. Alchemy presupposes that what we are given, and what we find in our surroundings, is the prima materia, the base material to be transformed. Now is the time to embrace our practices and our tools—whatever they are—diligently, prayerfully, and with intention. Those of us who are connected to spirit through guides can simply ask for direction. As more of us enter and dwell in the dimension of the heart, our hearts become the source of our guidance. As we carry the resonance of love into the world wherever we are and through whatever we do, the easier it will be for others to find compatibility and resonance in their own hearts.

Regardless of how you go about it—no matter what tools you choose to use or what discipline you choose to practice, the movement from Will to Heart is essential to the quality of our lives, both individually and collectively, in the future we are co-creating.

21
THE CRYSTAL
CAULDRON

THIS FINAL JOURNEY is the completion of the sacred Journey of Alchemical Healing. It presupposes that you have practiced the work that has been offered throughout this book, and that you have the capacity to remain heart-centered, fully present and conscious in the realm of Akasha. During this journey and in subsequent practice, you will receive information direct from source without personal or cultural filtration. To have access to Akasha in this way empowers you to tap directly the infinite potential of the creative process, its intelligence, its information, and its abilities to dissolve and rebuild. This journey will also provide a limitless supply of Akasha that you can use as a healing balm to relieve suffering anywhere you find it.

When you have become comfortable with this new way of accessing Akasha and have a clear sense of its potential and its effects, you can begin directing it from the endless supply available through your overflowing, continuously refilling, crystal cauldron. Initially repeat this journey as a practice. At some point it will take on a life of its own, issuing forth constantly, and informing you on how and when you need to use it. Soon you will have continuous access to this crystal cauldron within. Remember, Akasha requires that you be fully cognizant of your thoughts, emotions, and intentions, and centered within your heart.

JOURNEY
THE CRYSTAL CAULDRON

Be sure you have created sacred space and are appropriately prepared. . . . Close your eyes, ground and center. . . . Begin practicing the Heart Breath, and acknowledge the sigil from the card within. . . .

Place your hands before you and receive a new Akashic egg in your hands. . . .

Place the egg in your abdomen. . . .

Focus on your heart. Take a few moments to find the feeling of love, the emanations of compassion, peace, and serenity, and the untainted wisdom represented by Thoth that dwells in the glow of your heart, and sit with that for a few moments as your heart flame brightens and grows. . . .

Direct your attention to the crown at your seventh chakra, for this is the doorway through which you will draw down the magic of Akasha when it is time. . . .

Now bring your attention to where the egg has been gestating in your belly. As you observe the Akashic egg, it begins to dissolve in the primordial waters in your abdomen. It completely dissolves and mixes with the waters. Small crystals begin to form in the solution. Each crystal is a nucleus that attracts more of the crystalline molecules to precipitate out of the solution, and they begin to grow. As they find and connect with one another, a larger crystal takes shape, formed by all of the smaller crystals bonding together into the shape of a cauldron. . . .

This process continues until the liquids are completely clear, and a bright, luminous cauldron, a crystal cauldron, is nestled in your belly. It is sparkling, faceted, and clear—filled with the waters of life. At the end, as the final crystals come out of solution, the only remaining liquid is that which is within the cauldron. . . .

Notice a subtle fragrance, that of the herb rosemary. Offer a blessing of energy and love to the family of the rosemary plant and invite it into your cauldron. As the essence of the plant enters the cauldron and steeps in the primordial soup, the scent becomes stronger. . . .

Reach in and stir the waters of life within your crystal cauldron. The waters begin to rise. Streams of water snake upward to meet the flame in your heart. When the water enters the fire, it does not diminish it in any way. Steam explodes from this hissing and bubbling mix, and begins to spread throughout your body. The steam that is filling every part of you carries the essence of rosemary, which helps to facilitate memory. Use all your senses to perceive the steam moving through your body, energizing you. It enters your organs, your bones, your muscles, your cells. . . . It moves out through your shoulders and down through your arms and hands all the way to your fingertips. . . . It moves down through your pelvis, your hips and legs, down to your toes. . . . It moves up through your chest and throat, filling your head until it has permeated your entire being. The steam keeps on coming and moving through you until there is no more water left in the cauldron. It's as though you were boiling a kettle dry, but without harm. Smell the fragrance of the rosemary that has been released through the steam, and it will help you remember.

Give yourself time here. . . .

When the crystal cauldron is empty, it is time to draw down Akasha. Raise your hands above your head and draw the symbol of the vesica piscus to open the Akashic doorway. Reach through the symbol and pull down Akasha. . . . Notice how the cloud of purple-black fog pours down from above, enters through your crown, and fills your crystal cauldron. This seething, potent, roiling Akasha within your cauldron has an endless source.

It billows out to permeate your entire body. Remain as present as possible and pay close attention. The Akasha absorbs all of the memories that have been released by the rosemary, whether or not you are aware of them. It penetrates your entire inner being, absorbing and dissolving all aspects of the old paradigm that no longer serve you. Stay present within the Akasha and let it reveal to you its teachings for this time. There may be a message, a story, a journey, or an experience that will inform you about your true path. . . .

Allow as much time as it takes. . . .

If you are living with pain, this is an opportunity to direct some of that unlimited supply of Akasha to soothe and alleviate your pain. . . .

When your experience is complete, it is time for gratitude. Give thanks to Thoth, the rosemary, the crystal, the elements, and the mystery that provided this awakening. . . .

It is particularly important to ground yourself after working with Akasha. . . . Feel your connection to the earth and take the time you need to fully integrate your experience. . . . When you are ready, open your eyes.

Though it seems paradoxical, it is important to know that you can place yourself within this crystal cauldron that resides within yourself. Anytime you become confused or begin to doubt your truth, draw Akasha from the infinite source, and find peace within.

Warning: It's best not to practice this technique while driving.

★ ☽ ★

Your crystal cauldron has many uses:

- As a healing balm for you and for any person, place, or situation needing calm, soothing energies
- As a means of alleviating pain in yourself or another
- As a place to start over when you've been going down a path that is not serving you and you have run out of options (when nothing but complete dissolution is going to work, it's time for the crystal cauldron)
- As a comforter when you are drowning in grief
- As a calm, serene, and secure place to be when tidying up loose ends at the end of your life, or at the end of a major segment of your life
- As a place of joyous celebration of a decision to create new life, such as a child or a great work of art or endeavor

AFTERWORD
ALCHEMICAL GOLD

THE SACRED JOURNEY of Alchemical Healing has no end. My own long and winding passage is but a testimony to the possibilities of transformation, of lead into gold—and it is still, and most likely will always be, a work in progress. When viewed in the larger scheme of things, beyond the split second of a life lived passionately in a fraction of eternity, it is ultimately a journey with no final goal. "There is no end to becoming . . ." translates Normandi Ellis in *Awakening Osiris: The Egyptian Book of the Dead.* "The doors of perception open; what was hidden has been revealed. . . . As the houses of earth fill with dancing and song, so filled are the houses of heaven. I come, in truth. I sail a long river and row back again. It is joy to breathe under the stars. I am the sojourner destined to walk a thousand years until I arrive at myself."*

Each process given in these pages offers an opportunity to mine the rich resources of your inner landscape for the glint of gold, in the light of which wisdom dwells. Each healing to which these tools are directed extends the life of the knowledge, which is renewed moment by moment in the imagination of those who find and delight in these pages. To wrest purpose from our suffering, to trans-

---

*Normandi Ellis, *Awakening Osiris: The Egyptian Book of the Dead* (Grand Rapids, Mich.: Phanes Press, 1988), 220–221.

form our most adverse situations into our power, to make use of and find respect for the myriad obstacles and tests we encounter in our journey, is to refine and polish our personal philosophers' stone. After all, at the end of your life, what would you wish to leave behind?

Once you have completed all the exercises in this book, return to the chapter on commitment. Journey once again to Thoth to reiterate or establish a new level of commitment that honors the work you have done and the changes you have made.

"We are gods in the body of god, truth and love our destinies. Go then and make of the world something beautiful, set up a light in the darkness."*

---

*Ibid., 222.

APPENDIX I
THE EMERALD TABLET

THE FOLLOWING IS THE TEXT OF The Emerald Tablet, as translated by Dennis William Hauck in *The Emerald Tablet: Alchemy for Personal Transformation* (New York: Penguin Compass, 1999).

♦♦♦

In truth, without deceit, certain, and most veritable.

That which is Below corresponds to that which is Above, and that which is Above corresponds to that which is Below, to accomplish the miracles of the One Thing. And just as all things have come from this One Thing, through the meditation of One Mind, so do all created things originate from this One Thing, through Transformation.

Its father is the Sun; its mother the Moon. The Wind carries it in its belly; its nurse is the Earth. It is the origin of All, the consecration of the Universe; its inherent Strength is perfected, if it is turned into Earth.

Separate the Earth from Heaven, the Subtle from the Gross, gently and with great Ingenuity. It rises from Earth to Heaven and descends again to Earth, thereby combining within Itself the powers of both the Above and the Below.

Thus, will you obtain the Glory of the Whole Universe. All Obscurity will be clear to you. This is the greatest Force of all powers, because it overcomes every Subtle thing and penetrates every Solid thing.

In this way was the Universe created. From this comes many wondrous Applications, because this is the Pattern.

Therefore am I called Thrice Greatest Hermes, having all three parts of the wisdom of the Whole Universe. Herein have I completely explained the Operation of the Sun.

♦♦♦

APPENDIX II

AUTHORIZED ALCHEMICAL HEALING TEACHERS AND PRACTITIONERS

PROGRAMS ARE AVAILABLE for further studies of Alchemical Healing and related subjects. The following list is of those authorized to give initiation, activations, and empowerments in Alchemical Healing at the time of printing. If you are interested in deepening your studies or becoming a teacher, please contact the author directly, or any of those listed below.

ACTIVE AUTHORIZED TEACHERS AND PRACTITIONERS FROM THE LINEAGE:

U.S.A.

Active Teachers of Alchemical Healing

Nicki Scully
Eugene, OR
541-484-1099
800-937-2991
nscully@shamanicjourneys.com

Bo Clark
Cloudland, GA
HawksAbove@aol.com
www.HawksAbove.com

Kalita Todd Cantisano
PO Box 942
North San Juan, CA 95960
530-292-3610
kalitatodd@hotmail.com

Imani White
Rockville, MD
301-977-4547
mzimani@ctsgathering.net
www.ctsgathering.net

Danielle Hoffman
Seattle, WA
206-323-2762
dannihoffy@earthlink.net
www.remembertobreathe.com

Rev. Kathryn Ravenwood
PO Box 808
Tonasket, WA 98855
509-485-3912
kravenwood@yahoo.com

Gloria Taylor Brown
Seattle, WA
206-440-7311
gloria@alchemyarts.com

Charla Hermann
Valley Head, AL
256-635-6304
tarwater@vol.com

Greg Okulove
San Francisco, CA
Gokulove@aol.com

*Practioners and Other
Lineage Members*

David Groode
Intuitive consultant and
numerologist
Sebastapol, CA
707-824-8949
clayartist@aol.com

Chris Tice
Intuitive consultant
Occidental, CA
donchris@sonic.net

Bambi Merryweather, Ph.D.,
O.M.D., L.Ac.
Alchemical Healing/Chinese
Medicine
San Diego/San Francisco, CA
858-454-1487
sai108@aol.com

Paul Kervick
Monkton, VT
802-425-2346
paul@awakening sanctuary.org

Jane Bell
San Francisco, CA
jane@presenceofheart.com

Bobbie Holloway, CMT
Sonora, CA
bobbie@prescenceofheart.com

Janice Wilson
Portland, OR
janicejean3@attbi.com

Joan Porter
Alchemical Healing and Focusing
Portola Valley, CA
Stillheart316@aol.com

Mira Sophia
Ashland, OR
www.intothemystery.com

Normandi Ellis
PO Box 51
Frankfort, KY 40602
ellisisis@aol.com

Patricia Sell
Seattle, WA/Scottsdale, AZ
patcgsell@aol.com

Mark Hallert
Eugene, OR
www.mementos.net
Mementos@earthlink.net

EUROPE

Teachers and Practioners

Dr. Christine Fehling-Joss
Psychiatry and Psychotherapy,
FMH
Thunstrasse 40
Ch 3005 Bern, Switzerland
031-351-95-85
fehling-joss@tiscalinet.ch

Hiltrud (Anugama) Marg
Starklef 40
25938 Wyk, Föhr
Germany
046-81-74-80-78
Hiltrud.Marg@t-online.de

Pia Ammann
Thunstrasse 38
Ch 3005 Bern, Switzerland
031-352-91-67
ammann.pia@bluemail.ch

Erika Radermacher
Schaufelweg 26
CH-3098 Schliern/Bern,
Switzerland
031-971-04-65 or 079-699-70-60

Annemarie Staub
Schaeppi-Naefstr.8
Ch 8942 Oberrieden
Switzerland
031-720-25-77

Margrit Meier
Schaufelweg 26
CH-3098 Schliern/Bern
Switzerland
margrit.meier@bbw.admin.ch

INDEX

accidents, 164, 179–80
accountability, 188–89
Activating the Fire Mist Shower, 81–84
Air, 16
  and the chakras, 67–68
  description of, 106–7
  and music, 259–60
aka, 63, 111, 158
Akasha, 107–9, 207–10
  and advanced empowerment, 225–28
  and the Akashic Record, 215–16
  and the chakras, 68
  and DNA, 213–14
  for healing, 218–25
  and healing through time, 210–13
  and music, 260–61
  practice of, 216–17

alchemy, stages of, 10–15
allies, 171–72
altars, 56
anger, 268
animal totems. *See also* specific totems
  introduction to, 39–40
  relationships with, 121–25
  and removing disease, 160
  and shields, 171–72
Anubis, 129, 171–72
archetypes, 125–31
astrology, 99
attachment, 74
attention, 56, 76, 203, 296
auras and auric fields, 73, 75–76, 89, 152–54
Awakening the Cobra, 15
ayne, 184, 276

ALSO BY NICKI SCULLY

Shamanic Mysteries of Egypt
Awakening the Healing Power of the Heart
Bear & Company, 2007

Power Animal Meditations
Shamanic Journeys with Your Spirit Allies
Illustrated by Angela Werneke
Bear & Company, 2001

CDs Available from Nicki Scully

Journey for Healing with Kuan Yin
With music by Roland Barker and Jerry Garcia
Track One: Journey for Healing with Kuan Yin
Track two: Music only
Nicki Scully, 2006

Proceeds from the sale of this CD go toward the production
and distribution of more of these CDs to be given away to people
with AIDS, leukemia, or cancer, or to centers and practitioners
working with those diseases. Donations are tax deductible.

The first three of the following CDs can function as audio
illustrations for Power Animal Meditations

Awakening the Cobra
With music by Roland Barker
Track one: Journey with the Cobra for Clearing the
Chakras and Awakening the Kundalini Energies
Track two: Music only

Journey with Eagle & Elephant
With music by Roland Barker
Track one: Journey with Eagle & Elephant
Track two: Music only

Tribal Alchemy
Three journeys are available on this CD: Renewal, Journey
for Peace, and Animal Totems
Music produced and arranged by Roland Barker
Nicki Scully, 1996

. . . And You Will Fly!
An Animal Circus Adventure (for children of all ages)
Written by Nicki Scully, Roland Barker, and Mark Hallert
Narrated by Nicki Scully
Music written and produced by Roland Barker
Sahalie Publishing, 2001

An Alchemical healing story produced as a radio play
for children to be given away free to any child suffering
from a potentially terminal disease, and to those hospitals
and practitioners working with these children. Proceeds from
the sale of this CD will go toward further production and
distribution so that more can be given away.

To order, contact your local bookseller or
Nicki Skully
P.O. Box 5025
Eugene, OR 97405
www.shamanicjourneys.com
office@shamanicjourneys.com

BOOKS OF RELATED INTEREST

Power Animal Meditations
Shamanic Journeys with Your Spirit Allies
by Nicki Scully

The Anubis Oracle
A Journey into the Shamanic Mysteries of Egypt
by Nicki Scully and Linda Star Wolf

Shamanic Mysteries of Egypt
Awakening the Healing Power of the Heart
by Nicki Scully and Linda Star Wolf

Shamanic Breathwork
Journeying beyond the Limits of the Self
by Linda Star Wolf

The Temples of Light
An Initiatory Journey into the Heart Teachings
of the Egyptian Mystery Schools
by Danielle Rama Hoffman

Coyote Healing
Miracles in Native Medicine
by Lewis Mehl-Madrona, M.D., Ph.D.

Light: Medicine of the Future
How We Can Use It to Heal Ourselves NOW
by Jacob Liberman, O.D., Ph.D.

The Cherokee Full Circle
A Practical Guide to Ceremonies and Traditions
by J. T. Garrett and Michael Tlanusta Garrett

Inner Traditions • Bear & Company
P.O. Box 388
Rochester, VT 05767
1-800-246-8648
www.InnerTraditions.com

Or contact your local bookseller